VERSES KINDLER PUBLICATION

Medical Consents: Explained

- With special emphasis on UAE rules and regulations

Verses Kindler Publication

<u>DISCLAIMER</u>

Medical Consents: Explained - With special emphasis on UAE rules and regulations is written by Dr. Shaik Mohiuddin.

The published work is original content that has been carefully edited to ensure it is free of plagiarism.

It is important to note that this book is intended as general reading material and is not a substitute for staying informed about the latest developments in medical consent laws and regulations. While it provides a foundational understanding of the subject, readers are strongly urged to consult official sources for up-to-date information. It should be recognized that regulations governing medical consents can vary between regions and may be influenced by evolving ethical standards and legal precedents. It is crucial for readers to always consult with the latest laws and regulations on medical consents in their jurisdiction.

Medical professionals should regularly refer to the most recent laws and regulations established by relevant authorities in their jurisdiction. Seeking guidance from local medical associations can also provide valuable insight into best practices concerning obtaining informed consent from patients.

It is also important to note that any characters in this book may be fictitious or based on real events, but they are not intended to harm anyone's feelings or to portray anything against any caste or system.

The author is solely responsible for any plagiarized content in the write-up, and the publisher would not be held responsible for it.

<u>ACKNOWLEDGEMENT STATEMENT</u>

Before diving into the details of this comprehensive work on medical consents, it's important to express my deepest gratitude and appreciation to my mentors and those who have significantly influenced my life and career. I am profoundly grateful for the love, support, and encouragement I have received from my family, especially my wife and our wonderful children. Their unwavering belief in my abilities has been a constant source of motivation and inspiration.

Moreover, there is one individual whose influence on my life is unparalleled – my late father. His wisdom, guidance, and unwavering faith in me have left an indelible mark on my work ethic and thirst for knowledge. His sacrifices and guidance have shaped the person I am today and enabled me to embark on this writing journey. His legacy is a constant source of inspiration as I strive to honor him by contributing meaningfully to the field of healthcare quality and patient safety.

Table of Contents

CHAPTER 1: HISTORICAL CONTEXT OF CONSENT AND ITS BACKGROUND IN HEALTH CARE

The contemporary healthcare landscape has undergone a significant transformation due to the increasing emphasis on popular sovereignty, which is fundamentally rooted in the notion of governance by the consent of the governed. This shift in thought is exemplified by the English Civil War of the mid-seventeenth century, where a growing reaction against autocratic rule emerged. During this tumultuous period, the concept of the divine right of kings clashed with the idea of a parliament's authority, which was grounded in popular customs and consent. Sir Edward Coke, an influential figure during that era, made a compelling case for this shift, in a speech he delivered in parliament in 1621, stating that when the king claims the authority to deny our inherent liberties, it strikes at the very core of our society, as we represent the interests of thousands and tens of thousands of individuals. This marked a significant departure from the previous belief in the absolute authority of the monarchy.

Even notable proponents of monarchy, like Thomas Hobbes, acknowledged the centrality of individual consent in establishing sovereign authority. Hobbes, in his influential works, proposed that sovereign authority should be based on a covenant formed through the respective consent of each citizen, with monarchy being his preferred outcome of such a covenant. The American Revolutionary War also prominently featured the theme of political consent. The Declaration of Independence explicitly referred to the importance of consent, asserting that governments are established by men and derive their just powers from the consent of the governed. It is likely that John Locke's ideas on consent, as articulated in his "Two Treatises of Government," played a significant role in shaping this document. Locke's argument, particularly in contrast to Hobbes, offered a defence of the right to revolution when a government breaches its consensual contract with the people, a concept that resonated with the colonists. While Locke and Hobbes had differing degrees of boldness in their positions, both concurred that government by consent, grounded in a social contract, was compatible with various forms of governance, including monarchy and other non-democratic political structures.

Furthermore, the concept of consent transcends the realm of politics and extends into various aspects of our lives, especially in the context of medical interventions and patient rights. If we consider the absence of interference from others as a fundamental right, it becomes evident that consent plays a pivotal role in ensuring that actions are not coercive in nature. In this context, permissive consent, wherein the patient's right of choice is upheld irrespective of the reasons behind their decision, is seen as paramount. This perspective underscores the notion that individuals have the autonomy to make choices, whether those choices are rational, irrational, unknown, or even non-existent. Such a libertarian strand of liberalism has, however, faced fierce opposition, and the boundaries of consent remain subject to ongoing debate and clarification.

1.1 Early Concepts of Consent in Healthcare

In antiquity, health and wellness were often attributed to divine forces, with offerings, incantations, and amulets serving as conventional safeguards against afflictions. Nevertheless, a distinct cadre of healthcare practitioners emerged, postulating their capacity to provide solutions beyond the purview of the gods. This progression involved meticulous scrutiny of causative factors, manifestation of symptoms, and exploration of therapeutic interventions. Notably, philosophers ventured into the realm of medical theory, positing comprehensive elucidations of human physiology and the genesis of pathological imbalances.

Medical practitioners of yore were not only concerned with commonplace maladies but also extended their expertise to address wartime injuries and conduct intricate surgical procedures, including the enigmatic practice of trephination. This examination delves into the perspectives on health and medical practices in the ancient realms of Mesopotamia, Egypt, Greece, Additionally, the Greek deity of healing, Asclepius, and renowned physicians like Hippocrates, whose ethical code is known as the Hippocratic Oath. Till date, it continues to serve as a revered tenet embraced by contemporary medical practitioners worldwide.

Ancient medical practices have undergone a transformative evolution, encompassing peculiar methods and enduring concepts that are still integral to contemporary healthcare. This evolution spans centuries of diligent research, culminating in the establishment of what we now recognise as modern medicine.

A cornerstone of contemporary healthcare is the principle of informed consent, wherein healthcare providers meticulously educate patients about the inherent risks, advantages, and viable alternatives associated with a particular medical procedure or intervention. This process necessitates the patient's competency to make an autonomous and deliberate choice regarding their willingness to undergo the proposed medical course. Informed consent represents an ethical and legal imperative for medical practitioners in many parts of the world, stemming from a patient's fundamental right to dictate the course of their medical treatment.

Implicit within the provision of informed consent is a thorough assessment of the patient's comprehension, followed by the issuance of a well-informed recommendation and meticulous documentation of this process. The Joint Commission, a pivotal authority in healthcare dedicated to enhancing public health services, consistently mandates the thorough documentation of every facet of the informed consent discussion. This requirement extends to meticulous record-keeping, encompassing progress notes and integration within the patient's medical do̶c̶u̶m̶e̶n̶t̶ documentation encompasses the nature of the procedure, the associated risks and benefits, available alternatives, the potential risks and benefits of these alternatives, and a robust evaluation of the patient's comprehension of each element. This rigorous framework ensures that the sanctity of informed consent remains a central tenet of contemporary medical practice.

1.2 Historical Foundations of Consent

Historical landmarks in medical ethics reveal a conspicuous absence of the fundamental principle of informed consent, as evidenced by seminal works such as the Hippocratic writings from the fifth to fourth century B.C. and Thomas Percival's "Medical Ethics" in 1803. These revered documents predominantly focused on shielding patients from distressing information, emblematic of an era when medical ethics primarily adhered to non-disclosure. The concept of informed consent was subsequently introduced into the medical field via external avenues of authority, notably judges in legal settings and government officials overseeing regulatory agencies.

The transformation towards a duty to secure consent, particularly in surgical procedures, began during the 1950s and 1960s. This evolution originated in the courtroom and culminated in an explicit obligation to divulge specific information and secure consent, both in clinical practice and research. It was during this period that the term "informed consent" emerged, first appearing in the landmark legal decision of Salgo v. Leland Stanford, Jr. University Board of Trustees in 1957. In this pioneering case, the court posited that disclosing risks and treatment alternatives did not establish a novel obligation but rather an inherent extension of the preexisting duty to reveal the nature and consequences of medical intervention. Salgo thus marked the genesis of the informed consent doctrine by emphasising not only the mere presence of consent but also its essential requirement of being adequately informed.

Following this momentous development, a succession of court cases incrementally introduced additional obligations into the framework of informed consent. The post-Salgo era was characterised by gradual legal changes, which lasted for about fifteen years. Then, a watershed moment occurred in 1972 when three separate state courts in the United States delivered groundbreaking decisions that would elevate the moral and legal significance of informed consent. The pivotal cases were Canterbury v. Spence, Cobbs v. Grant, and Wilkinson v. Vesey. Among them, Canterbury exerted a profound influence by advocating for a more patient-centric standard of disclosure. Judge Spottswood Robinson articulated that "the patient's right to self-determination delineates the boundaries of disclosure duty.

This right can only be meaningfully exercised when the patient possesses adequate information to make an informed choice." Consequently, informed consent not only retained its legal standing but also assumed a more substantial role, encompassing ethical considerations in both medical practice and research.

The aftermath of these legal milestones witnessed a surge in medical literature exploring issues related to informed consent, with a particular emphasis on the impact of precedent-setting cases. Physicians expressed concerns about the potential rise in malpractice risks associated with this newfound legal dimension, prompting extensive discussions in the medical community. A study conducted in the mid-1960s by a collaborative team of lawyers and surgeons revealed that consent forms were not yet a commonplace feature, even within the realm of surgical practice, let alone other medical disciplines. However, the landscape rapidly transformed following the 1972 court decisions.

The years between 1972 and 1978 marked a remarkable consolidation of the belief that physicians and biomedical researchers shared both a moral and legal obligation to obtain consent for specific medical procedures. These developments triggered a proliferation of critical commentary within the medical literature during the mid-1970s. Physicians began to perceive the demands of informed consent as potentially unattainable and, in some instances, at odds with the principles of optimal patient care. These multifaceted ethical considerations posed a challenge for medical professionals as they navigated the evolving landscape of informed consent.

1.3 Enlightenment Era and the Birth of Modern Medicine

The notion of autonomy, which had an antiquated political connotation, experienced a significant transformation during the Enlightenment era. This period marked a profound shift in political, philosophical, social, and religious landscapes, characterised by overthrowing monarchies, dismantling hierarchical structures, and diminishing the influence of religious authorities. The resultant secularism confronted the formidable task of reconstructing and justifying ethical principles in the absence of divine guidance, thus posing a severe threat to social cohesion. In this context, the concept of autonomy evolved from being exclusively political to encompassing personal autonomy, a development attributed to the renowned philosopher and political theorist Jean-Jacques Rousseau.

The dark shadow cast by the Third Reich during and before World War II remains a chilling reminder of the ethical dilemmas within the field of medicine. The Doctors' Trials, conducted from 1946 to 1947 as part of the Subsequent Nuremberg Trials, revealed the heinous atrocities allegedly committed in the name of scientific research. The Nuremberg Code (N.C.) was meticulously crafted in response to these atrocities. Its opening statement underscored the utmost importance of securing the voluntary consent of human subjects, laying the foundation for what would evolve into the field of bioethics. Notably, Perley et al. (as cited in Annas and Grodin) elucidate that, within a mere decade of N.C.'s adoption, it directly and profoundly influenced the development of other pivotal ethical codes. Among these, the Declaration of Geneva (1948) and guidelines concerning N.C. principles, such as the doctrine of informed consent, were profoundly shaped by the principles enshrined in the Nuremberg Code.

Throughout the development of modern medical practices, ethical considerations have played a pivotal role in shaping the ethical framework governing medical research and practice. The evolution of autonomy, from its political origins to its contemporary embodiment as personal autonomy, reflects the intricate interplay between history, philosophy, and medicine in the pursuit of ethical healthcare practices.

1.4 19th Century and the Rise of Medical Professionalism

Prior to the late 1950s, the concept of informed consent lacked a solid foundation within the field of medicine. It is crucial to acknowledge that, throughout history, both prominent figures in ancient, medieval, and modern medicine have addressed issues of information management in their interactions with patients and research subjects. Nevertheless, a comprehensive history of these interactions, as it pertains to informed consent, is somewhat unsatisfactory. Delving into the annals of medical ethics, one encounters the Hippocratic Corpus, a classic text from ancient medicine, which predominantly emphasises a physician's duty to deliver medical benefits to patients and safeguard them from harm. The essence of treatment, as outlined in the Hippocratic oath, was rooted in the betterment of the sick and the prevention of hurt and injustice. Within this context, handling information in patient interactions was predominantly depicted as a matter of prudence and discretion, with no explicit emphasis on the obligation of truthfulness.

It is worth noting that in the nineteenth century, a notable exception to the prevailing consensus on medical disclosure emerged, primarily supported by Connecticut physician Worthington Hooker. Hooker marked the onset of a shift towards recognising the rights of patients to be informed, opposing the long-standing model of benevolent deception that had been upheld from the era of Hippocrates to the American Medical Association (AMA). In addition to Hooker, Harvard professor of medicine Richard Clarke Cabot also contributed to this emerging perspective prior to the latter half of the twentieth century. Nevertheless, even within Hooker's novel and ingenious arguments, one cannot find an explicit endorsement of informed consent. His primary concern lies in addressing the deleterious impact of deception on society and the integrity of medical institutions rather than advocating for obtaining patients' consent or respecting their autonomy for its own sake. Hooker's arguments centred on the expediency of disclosure and truth-telling rather than promoting autonomous decision-making or the concept of informed consent. The idea that patients should possess a comprehensive understanding of their medical condition to participate in treatment decisions actively was a notion yet to develop within the medical community fully.

1.5 20th Century and Legal Landmarks

The notion of informed consent within the medical context has a relatively recent origin, tracing its roots to a series of four legal judgments in the early 20th century that laid the foundational principles of patient autonomy. The evolution of legal obligations regarding disclosure and the right of patients to self-determination unfolded progressively. In the realm of legal precedent, each decision, drawing from earlier court rulings, becomes part of an authoritative chain that incorporates pertinent language and rationale from the cited cases. Consequently, a small number of initial consent-related cases gradually converged into a legal doctrine. Among these early cases, Schloendorff v. New York Hospital (1914) stands out as the most renowned and influential. Schloendorff utilised the concept of self-determination to justify the imposition of an obligation to seek a patient's consent. Subsequent cases that followed and referenced Schloendorff implicitly embraced its justificatory framework. Thus, the principle of self-determination emerged as the primary rationale underpinning the legal imperative for obtaining patient consent.

During the early 20th century, physicians' conduct often exhibited egregious lapses, and the courts did not shy away from using unequivocal language and sweeping principles to condemn such behaviour. This same language subsequently served as a legal precedent in cases where physicians' actions were less flagrant. As the doctrine of informed consent continued to evolve and confront more nuanced issues, the legal framework could have deviated from the concept of self-determination. However, it instead increasingly relied on this foundational premise. The language employed in the early cases strongly suggests that the right to be free from bodily intrusion inherently encompasses the rights of patients to make informed medical decisions.

The Nuremberg Military Tribunal's verdict in the case of the United States v Karl Brandt et al. stands as a seminal moment in the annals of medical ethics, bestowing upon the world the Nuremberg Code. This decalogue of principles, enshrined within the tribunal's decision, delineates the parameters for ethically permissible medical experimentation on human subjects. According to this codified doctrine, the sanctity of humane investigation is predicated upon its capacity to yield societal benefits while adhering to fundamental tenets that unequivocally "satisfy moral, ethical, and legal concepts."

This landmark declaration, situated within the context of Nuremberg between October 1946 and April 1949, represents a critical juncture in the evolution of medical ethics. Its overarching message underscores the imperative of aligning medical research with moral and legal precepts, affirming that scientific progress must be harmoniously wedded to ethical standards.

However, in the contemporary landscape of medical research, challenges persist in the realm of data-sharing and patient-controlled Data Sharing Ecosystems (DSE). Notably, legal constraints are only one of the impediments to achieving seamless DSE. Additional constraints manifest in the form of investigators' ambitions to publish their findings expeditiously, along with the interests of research funders. A more lucid regulatory framework can ameliorate this impediment, facilitating the unhindered operation of robust DSE systems, ideally controlled by patients themselves.

In this context, the International Clinical Trial Center Network (ICN), a consortium uniting the expertise of 19 clinical trial centres across the globe, plays a pivotal role. This network offers a simplified overview of the regulatory prerequisites for the exchange of health data and biospecimens across four continents, illuminating disparities that could influence the execution of international projects. The ICN unites various non-profit institutions with a shared mission of fostering ongoing international discourse, providing guidance to researchers, and promoting global collaboration. Furthermore, it scrutinises pertinent terms relating to data protection. This collaborative endeavour holds the potential to advance the global exchange of data and biospecimens, serving as a valuable resource for researchers engaged in large-scale international research initiatives.

1.6 Contemporary Perspectives on Consent in Healthcare

Consent is undeniably regarded as the cornerstone of contemporary medical ethics and a pinnacle of ethical clinical practice. Central to the concept of consent is the principle that patients possess the capacity to make autonomous decisions, thus safeguarding themselves against potential harm. The validity of consent hinges upon the provision of comprehensive information to patients concerning any proposed clinical course, encompassing its alternatives, benefits, and associated risks.

In certain domains of medicine, the nexus between information disclosure and the preservation of patient autonomy is more lucidly delineated. This clarity arises from a direct alignment with the specific care objectives for an individual patient at a given moment. Consider, for instance, a surgical procedure characterised by a well-defined commencement and conclusion. Patients can be duly apprised of the procedural advantages, associated risks, and alternative options, empowering them to make an informed, autonomous decision.

Conversely, in other facets of medicine, the contours of the action necessitating consent are less defined, and therein lies an ongoing discourse amongst scholars and healthcare professionals (HCPs). This discourse pertains to the nature and extent of information required to attain a threshold of adequate consent while simultaneously preserving patient autonomy, mainly when the objectives of care may be less clearly demarcated.

1.7 Ethical Dilemmas and Future Trends

1. Mitigating Conflicts of Interest: Healthcare professionals, including doctors and nurses, often find themselves in the crosshairs of marketing efforts by pharmaceutical, medical device, and equipment manufacturers. To mitigate such influences, numerous organisations have implemented protocols requiring physicians to disclose conflicts of interest, including transparent reporting of financial contributions and gifts received by the institution. This establishes rigorous ethical standards, ensuring that physicians make patient-centered decisions devoid of any influence from pharmaceutical or marketing affiliations

2. Navigating the Conundrum of Equitable Treatment: The issue of ensuring equal treatment versus affording VIP privileges to donors and influential figures poses a significant ethical challenge. VIP patients, which may encompass financial donors and trustees' family members, demand particular attention. This can manifest as expedited waiting times, extended physician consultations, or direct involvement of hospital administrators to guarantee a superlative care experience.

3. Handling Patients with Diminished Decision-Making Capacity: When faced with paediatric and geriatric patients lacking total decision-making capacity, healthcare providers confront the arduous task of evaluating the patient's comprehension of their medical condition, the benefits and drawbacks of available

treatment options, and the potential consequences of opting for no treatment at all.

4. Mitigating Nurses' Moral Distress: A fundamental ethical challenge arises as nurses contend with moral distress resulting from providing care with limited medical benefit or a reduced quality of life for patients. Numerous nurses face the taxing responsibility of tending to patients on prolonged life support amid constrained resources and workplace pressures, which burdens them with the additional task of scrutinizing consent procedures. The deficiency in time allocation hampers the thorough identification of procedural inadequacies during the auditing process.

1.8 Global Perspectives on Healthcare Consent

Consent, an integral concept in health law, hinges upon the provision of comprehensive information pertaining to a patient's health condition and their entitlement to a full disclosure of all pertinent aspects of a proposed medical intervention. This disclosure stands at the core of an individual's capacity to make an informed choice. Informed consent, a legal instrument, is devised to safeguard personal autonomy and guard against arbitrary medical decisions. The understanding of informed consent remains a subject of ongoing refinement, embracing diverse interpretations on a global scale. Contemporary challenges persist, suggesting that unresolved issues impede a comprehensive grasp and application of this concept, both within national borders and on an international stage. This book embarks on a thorough exploration of this fundamental right, scrutinising it through various comparative lenses. It delves into the advantages signposted by the concept's evolution for patient rights and also contemplates the persisting challenges that hinder patients and the medical community alike.

The patient's entitlement to choose is firmly rooted in the ethical principle of autonomy or self-determination. Underpinning this moral precept, informed consent encapsulates the patient's right to make independent decisions concerning diagnosis and treatment following the receipt of all requisite information from the healthcare provider.

CHAPTER 2: DEFINITION OF CONSENT

Consent is the voluntary agreement of one individual to another's proposal or desires, a term commonly encountered in fields like law, medicine, research, and sexual relationships. In specific domains, the concept of consent may deviate from its everyday interpretation. For instance, obtaining patient consent for treatment is regarded as a crucial component in the provision of medical care. On numerous occasions, it is a simple undertaking, but in particular situations, it can be intricate and demanding to attain. Extensive deliberation on the matter has taken place, considering a multitude of ethical, religious, and legal viewpoints. Nonetheless, there are certain perspectives that require additional investigation and clarification. The different consent forms encompass implied, express, informed, and unanimous consent.

2.1 Fundamentals of Consent

Consent is a fundamental concept in the medical field, as well as in other domains. It is comprised of several essential elements. Firstly, consent should be freely given, devoid of any coercion or duress. Secondly, it necessitates complete comprehension, known as informed consent, which ensures that the consenting party clearly understands the implications of their decision. Thirdly, consent is specific, granted for a particular action or purpose. Fourthly, it is revocable, allowing individuals to withdraw their consent at any time. Lastly, consent must be continuous, meaning it's an ongoing process, not a one-time grant. These core components of consent hold great significance, particularly in the medical field, where they are crucial for safeguarding individual autonomy and rights.

Informed Consent: Informed consent is a fundamental process in the healthcare field, wherein a healthcare provider is responsible for imparting comprehensive information to a patient concerning the course of action, potential risks, advantages, and alternative courses of activity associated with a particular medical procedure or intervention. It is worth noting that while informed consents require disclosure of potential risks associated with a particular treatment or procedure, they also require disclosure of potential risks that may arise from not pursuing such treatment. It is essential to consider all the potential outcomes before arriving at any decision. Crucially, it mandates that the patient possess the capacity to autonomously decide whether to proceed with the procedure or intervention.

Administering treatment without a patient's consent is permissible only in emergency medical situations where immediate intervention is vital and obtaining consent is impossible due to the urgency or if the patient poses a risk to public health due to a contagious disease. Informed consent exemption applies when treating an unconscious patient whose benefits of treatment outweigh potential harm. In this case, the physician can treat the patient without obtaining informed consent but should do so as soon as medically possible. Regarding examinations, diagnoses, and initial medication dosage, consent from an incapacitated patient is considered valid if their family or designated representatives are informed of the treatment plan. Most regulators publish clear guidelines for consent procedures in such situations, like informing next of kin or a family member as prescribed by the jurisdictions in the region of your practice. Emergency treatment withholding or cessation of ongoing care is justifiable solely when patients defy medical guidance or due to uncontrollable circumstances, per

Articles (9) and (10) of this Decree-Law of the UAE Federal Law. Even then, physicians must seek the patient's consent for leaving against medical advice. This ensures adherence to legal provisions, maintaining ethical standards in healthcare delivery. The protocol underscores the importance of patient autonomy while safeguarding medical practitioners' responsibilities within the prescribed legal framework.

Voluntary Consent: Voluntary consent in medical treatment refers to the fundamental principle wherein an individual possesses the autonomy and sole authority to determine whether they wish to grant a specific medical intervention. This critical concept underscores the importance of respecting an individual's capacity for independent decision-making, free from undue influence, coercion, or persuasion exerted by healthcare practitioners, friends, or family members. It ensures that the individual's rights and choices remain central in medical decision-making.

Capacity and Competence: In the context of medical ethics, an essential consideration lies in the assessment of a patient's capacity and competence to provide informed consent. This pivotal process, central to medical practice, necessitates a meticulous evaluation of an individual's ability to comprehend relevant medical information, appreciate the potential risks and benefits of proposed interventions, and autonomously decide on their care. Profound emphasis is placed on safeguarding patient autonomy and ensuring the highest standard of care delivery, assessing capacity, a critical step in the ethical delivery of medical treatment.

Understanding, comprehension, and revocability within the context of medical consent hold prominent importance in the medical field. It delineates the necessity for patients to possess a clear and thorough grasp of the medical information provided, ensuring they can make informed decisions. Furthermore, it underscores the significance of patients having the right to revoke their consent at any point in the medical process if circumstances or their preferences change, upholding the ethical principles of autonomy and informed decision-making in medical treatment.

Obtaining valid consent is crucial before starting any treatment, even if other team members have already seen the patient. Documenting the discussions with patients in the process of gaining consent is essential. Patients have the right to know about the options for treatment, their risks, potential benefits, and the consequences. They can withdraw consent at any time. Written consent is necessary for treatment involving conscious sedation or general anaesthesia.

2.2 Principles Associated with Obtaining Consent

Adhering to the fundamental tenet of patient autonomy, it is incumbent upon healthcare practitioners to provide comprehensive and essential medical information, along with an array of available treatment alternatives. This ethical obligation facilitates the patient's ability to make informed decisions, fostering self-determination and upholding the principles of informed consent, veracity in communication, and safeguarding patient confidentiality.

The righteous principles of beneficence and non-maleficence are crucial in acquiring informed consent within the medical field. Beneficence involves the responsibility of healthcare professionals to enhance the patient's well-being by ensuring that proposed medical interventions offer potential advantages. Conversely, non-maleficence obliges them to prevent harm and minimize the associated risks of medical procedures. A harmonious equilibrium between these principles necessitates a comprehensive risk-benefit assessment and effective communication. It is noteworthy that contemporary medical advancements frequently give rise to intricate ethical quandaries, necessitating careful deliberations between innovation and patient welfare. Throughout this complex landscape, informed consent maintains its pivotal role as a safeguard.

The principles of justice and fairness also play a crucial role in the medical field, particularly concerning establishing informed consent. Justice necessitates ensuring equal access to healthcare resources and an unbiased approach to decision-making, eliminating discrimination based on age, gender, or socioeconomic status. The requirement for informed consent extends beyond ethical considerations; it is a legal mandate in most jurisdictions. A landmark example is the Nuremberg Code, crafted in the aftermath of World War II, which emphasized the significance of voluntary and informed consent in human experimentation. This code has set a global standard for ethical medical research, highlighting the dual nature of securing justice and fairness in consent procedures as both a moral and legal obligation with historical precedence.

Truthfulness and honesty are pivotal in obtaining informed consent in medical and scientific endeavours. Ensuring individuals fully understand a procedure or study's nature, risks, and benefits fosters autonomy and ethical research. Inaccurate information can lead to misguided decisions, undermining the integrity of healthcare and research. Transparent communication is essential, aligning with principles of bioethics and scientific integrity. Fostering a culture of veracity upholds ethical standards and empowers individuals to make informed choices, ultimately advancing the frontiers of medical and scientific knowledge.

In medical and scientific realms, upholding confidentiality and respecting privacy is a fundamental imperative while obtaining consent. It is paramount to assure patients and research participants that their personal information and data will be regulated with superior care and safeguarded. This unwavering commitment aligns with ethical standards and plays a pivotal role in building trust and encouraging individuals to engage in crucial medical and scientific activities. Implementing adequate safeguards, such as robust data encryption and secure storage protocols, fortifies the protection of sensitive information. As a result, this approach facilitates the responsible and safe advancement of knowledge in the medical and scientific fields. Therefore, it is unequivocal that confidentiality and privacy serve as the cornerstone of informed consent, ensuring the preservation of individual rights and upholding the integrity of research and healthcare practices.

2.3 Types of Consent in Healthcare

Implied Consent: Implied consent, as a concept, arises when an individual's participation in a particular circumstance is construed as an indication of their support. Where anonymity is diligently maintained, this practice finds reasonable acceptance, particularly in opinion surveys. However, its relevance may not extend seamlessly to marketing endeavours. Stringent privacy regulations, notably within the European Union, mandate marketers to obtain either explicit opt-in or opt-out consent from individuals. Relying on "implied consent" in these situations might lead to non-compliance with existing regulatory standards unless specific exemptions exist. For instance, a patient's agreement to undergo an examination in an outpatient setting is often seen as an implicit form of consent, however, as a requirement, healthcare organizations ensure a general consent is obtained from the patient to cover out patient and non-invasive care . In the UAE, the law requires a general consent that covers non-invasive clinical procedures, such as medical examinations and diagnostics.

Explicit Consent: Explicit Consent, or direct or express consent, denotes a scenario where an individual is provided with a clear choice regarding whether to grant permission for the collection, utilization, and potential sharing of their personal information before such data is gathered. This form of consent is mandated by worldwide privacy regulations whenever an organization intends to process a consumer's data, relying on consent as a legitimate legal basis. Essential components of explicit consent encompass the transparent and documented disclosure of the specifics pertaining to data collection and its intended purpose. It is noteworthy that explicit consent can be furnished through both written and verbal means, ensuring the utmost clarity and accountability.

Active Consent: Active consent in the medical context entails a consumer receiving a distinct statement, to which they must respond affirmatively, thereby indicating their permission through an active and explicit affirmation. This approach plays a crucial role in guaranteeing explicit and absolute consent in medical engagements. Within healthcare, consents remain active for a standard duration, typically 30 days, unless alterations to the treatment plan, withdrawal by the patient himself or herself, or shifts in the patient's condition warrant a revision.

Passive Consent: Passive consent represents an implied agreement in which the individual is presumed to have provided consent unless they explicitly express their objection. This approach may not align with the standards of organizations striving to adhere to privacy regulations that necessitate explicit consent.

Opt-out Consent: Opt-out consent refers to the essential capacity for individuals to withhold their consent at any given juncture. Consider, for instance, a scenario where an individual visits a website that provides an explicit option to decline consent. If the consumer chooses to proceed without an apparent refusal of consent, their acquiescence is effectively granted. It is noteworthy that this mode of support is typically documented in a written format.

2.4 Consent and Minors

The age of consent denotes the legally recognized threshold at which an individual is deemed capable of providing legal consent for engaging in sexual activities. Consequently, if an adult engages in sexual activity with a person below the age of consent, they cannot assert that the engagement was consensual from a legal standpoint. Such conduct may be classified as child sexual abuse or statutory rape. The individual falling under the stipulated minimum age is regarded as the victim and their sexual partner as the offender unless specific "Romeo and Juliet laws" are in place in certain jurisdictions, which offer exemptions when both participants are underage and of similar age.

Before going ahead with the procedure, it is necessary that there is proper consent, from both sides, that is the husband and the wife. The couple must be officially married and the hospital may demand a valid marriage certificate before the IVF. Furthermore, the couple must acquire a medical certificate from their physician which guarantees that both the mother and the foetus will not have any danger from ART (Assisted Reproductive Therapy). International rules and regulations for IVF may require different documentation as per their state policies.

In accordance with DHA and UAE Liability law on age, the guidelines for medical consent vary based on specific age brackets. Generally, individuals aged 18 and above are presumed as individuals capable of consenting to medical treatment without parental involvement unless they lack competence.

Emancipation is the legal procedure through which an individual below the age of 18, commonly referred to as a minor, attains the legal status of an adult. This status endows emancipated minors with the ability to provide informed consent for or deny medical treatments without the necessity of parental consent or notification. The route to emancipation varies by jurisdiction and may include factors such as child marriage, achieving financial self-sufficiency, acquiring an educational degree or diploma, or engaging in military service. In the United States, all states have established legal mechanisms for the emancipation of minors. In certain instances, emancipation can occur even without a formal court proceeding, with certain jurisdictions recognizing a minor as emancipated when they need to make decisions independently due to the absence of their parents or guardians. For instance, a minor in most jurisdictions can enter into legally binding contracts to secure their necessities. Nonetheless, in situations where parental provision is lacking, the child is often deemed a ward of the state, necessitating the appointment of a court-appointed guardian.

In the medical sphere, parental consent and notification refer to the legal obligations governing minors' access to healthcare services. The DHA and UAE laws stipulate that individuals under 18 are minors requiring parental or guardian consent for medical treatments. Healthcare providers, including DHA facilities, must obtain explicit consent from parents or legal guardians before administering care to minors. Failure to do so can result in legal repercussions due to violating patient consent laws. This ensures that minors' medical decisions align with their guardians' or parents' wishes and emphasizes the importance of respecting age-related consent regulations in healthcare settings to uphold legal and ethical standards. In addition DHA prescribes a sequence of priorities for consenting in case of minors.

2.5 Fertility Treatment Laws

The recent amendments in the Fertility Treatment Law in the United Arab Emirates have marked a significant turning point for married couples aspiring to undergo assisted reproductive technology (ART) procedures. Previously, the legislation in the UAE restricted the freezing and storage of embryos, compelling Emirati and international couples seeking IVF treatment to freeze only unfertilized oocytes and sperm. Consequently, many had to explore options abroad if they intended to preserve embryos for future cycles, rather than initiating IVF procedures anew. However, the updated ART law in the UAE has revolutionized this landscape by allowing the vitrification and storage of fertilized eggs (embryos) for future IVF cycles, marking an unprecedented shift in policy. This progressive adjustment empowers couples by permitting the preservation of embryos, necessitating only approval from the UAE's Ministry of Health to safeguard embryos and the couple's explicit written consent for storage in a cryobank.

Furthermore, the scope of these changes extends to gamete freezing and storage, enabling unmarried men and women to freeze their eggs or sperm for a period of five years, with the possibility of extending storage duration upon request. This development stands as a crucial stride in fertility preservation, particularly benefiting individuals undergoing medical treatments that affect fertility and those opting to marry at later stages in life.

The revised ART law delineates the eligibility criteria for individuals seeking fertility treatment in the UAE. Married couples, both Emirati and international, are eligible to apply for various fertility treatments, including IVF procedures. However, singles may only apply for egg or sperm freezing and storage, not for IVF treatment. Conversely, singles intending to undergo IVF with egg or sperm donation, along with non-married couples, are ineligible for fertility treatment in the UAE. The prerequisites for patient eligibility encompass several factors, including a minimum duration of attempting conception, infertility diagnosis affecting either or both partners, mutual consent for IVF treatment, official marriage certification, and medical certification attesting the safety of ART procedures for both the wife and potential fetus.

Under the purview of existing legislation, eligible couples can pursue a range of fertility treatments and other universally accepted fertilization techniques determined by the Oversight and Control Committee. However, specific treatments like using donor gametes for IVF, gestational surrogacy, traditional surrogacy, and preimplantation genetic diagnosis are prohibited by law. Furthermore, the revised law outlines procedures for cryopreservation, specifying conditions for the storage, disposal, and destruction of embryos, unfertilized oocytes, and sperm. Importantly, the law prohibits the commercial use of gametes and embryos without explicit consent and prohibits their use for scientific research without the couple's written authorization.

Current legislation in the UAE permits Emirati and foreign couples to access specific fertility treatments. These include IUI (Intrauterine Insemination) using the husband's sperm, GIFT (Gamete Intrafallopian Transfer), ZIFT (Zygote Intrafallopian Transfer), IVF (In Vitro Fertilization) using the wife's oocytes and the husband's sperm, and IVF–ICSI (Intracytoplasmic Sperm Injection). Additionally, any widely recognized fertilization methods can be considered, subject to a Cabinet decision proposed by the Oversight and Control Committee. The new legislation also addresses the logistics of shipping eggs and sperm, permitting the transportation of frozen gametes between clinics, subject to specific controls and procedures previously restricted under the older law. Nevertheless, the transfer of gametes between clinics necessitates the couple's written consent and approval from the Health Authority.

These recent amendments in the Fertility Treatment Law in the UAE signify a monumental shift, allowing greater reproductive freedom and options for married couples and individuals seeking fertility preservation. These regulatory changes not only broaden the scope of available treatments but also emphasize the importance of ethical considerations and consent for infertility-related procedures within the country. .

2.6 Challenges and Ethical Considerations in Obtaining Consent

The informed consent process originates in a societal movement that seeks to empower individuals and grant them greater autonomy. It also emerged in response to life-saving medical advancements, which sometimes raised questions about the perceived value of specific treatments. In medical care, informed consent assumes a pivotal role, with the patient and healthcare provider actively formulating a medically acceptable plan. Ethical obligations that underscore the importance of promoting autonomy, providing comprehensive information, and avoiding unethical biases are central to this process.

Patients possess the unequivocal right to decline medical therapies, whether grounded in religious convictions or other legitimate reasons, provided they have the requisite competence to make such decisions. Moreover, healthcare providers are unequivocally prohibited from subjecting patients to specific perioperative tests without obtaining informed consent. Furthermore, the principle of inclusivity prevails, ensuring that all patients, regardless of age, should be actively engaged in the medical decision-making process to the extent their capacity allows.

Within the framework of human research, a triad of responsibilities exists, namely, the investigator, the sponsor, and the Institutional Review Board, all of whom share the duty to safeguard the rights and welfare of research subjects. This entails thoroughly examining the fundamental components of informed consent and the procedural steps to be followed when securing such consent. Moreover, the circumstances under which the requirement for informed consent can be waived are scrutinized. Furthermore, physicians grapple with complex ethical dilemmas when obtaining informed consent from research subjects.

Requisites For Securing Informed Consent for Research:

In obtaining informed consent, it is imperative that either the investigator or a designated representative duly carry out this responsibility. Informed consent must be procured before any non-routine screening procedures are conducted or before modifying the subject's current medical regimen for the explicit purpose of a clinical trial. Importantly, no issue or their legally acceptable representative should ever be coerced into signing a consent form or be compelled to participate or continue participation in the trial. Moreover, it is incumbent upon both the subject or their legally acceptable representative and the individual responsible for obtaining consent to personally affix their signatures, accompanied by the date, to the consent form. These signatures testify to the comprehensive discussion of the informed consent document and the voluntary nature of the consent provided.

Challenges Encountered In The Informed Consent Process:

Language Barriers: One prominent challenge in the informed consent process pertains to language barriers. It is typically assumed that individuals who affix their signatures to consent forms fully comprehend the contents therein. However, evaluating the extent of a participant's comprehension of the provided information remains a formidable task due to the need for standardized methods for assessing this. Consequently, misunderstandings often arise, frequently attributable to incorrect translations of the document. Many individuals, unable to grasp the full import of what they are signing, may subsequently withdraw from ongoing clinical studies. Thus, when dealing with subjects from diverse linguistic backgrounds, the burden on researchers to ensure comprehensive understanding is heightened.

Religious Influence: Religious beliefs can significantly impact an individual's decision to participate in research projects. Frequently, experiment methodologies clash with the behavioural norms dictated by a participant's religious convictions. Consequently, religious considerations must be thoughtfully integrated into the informed consent process. In the case of an incompetent patient or a minor, informed consent can also be obtained from their legal guardian or next of kin. Here, the legal guardian or next of kin can demand a rightful explanation of the consent. However, if the minor doesn't have a legal guardian or next of kin, the consent of the most responsible physician can be considered. This must further be supervised by another healthcare professional.

Family: In matters concerning medical procedures or treatments associated with reproductive health, a married woman has the autonomy to provide her own Informed Consent, except where such procedures directly relate to her reproductive health. In the Emirates Law, In these specific instances, the consent of her husband takes precedence, prioritized over the consent of her father or legal guardian. This practice ensures due consideration for familial involvement in decisions concerning sensitive matters of reproductive healthcare.

False Expectations: Even when language barriers and religious considerations do not impede communication between researchers and participants, misunderstandings can persist due to participants' misconceptions about the expected outcomes of the experiment. Some patients fear being treated as mere "experimental subjects," while others are hesitant to participate due to historical instances of clinical trial fraud and misconduct. Managing these false expectations remains a critical challenge in the informed consent process.

Patient Perceptions: A prevalent concern among patients is the perceived burden of clinical trials. Many believe that conventional treatments are superior, while they harbour apprehensions about the unknown side effects associated with new therapies. Convincing such patients to provide informed consent is an intricate task. Striking a balance between providing adequate information about potential side effects and avoiding unnecessary deterrence from potentially life-saving or life-enhancing procedures is a delicate art in the informed consent process.

Vulnerable Individuals and Groups: Certain individuals and groups are inherently vulnerable, as they may lack the capacity to protect their interests. This vulnerability is particularly evident in individuals with learning disabilities. Their challenges in comprehending the nature of research, their role within it, and the implications of their participation necessitate special attention. Consequently, obtaining informed consent in such cases is especially complex, demanding tailored strategies for effectively conveying the ramifications of their involvement in research initiatives.

CHAPTER 3: TYPES OF CONSENT

3.1 Implied Consent

Implied consent, in contrast to express consent, where consent is overtly and unambiguously granted through explicit verbal communication, refers to consent inferred from a person's actions, gestures, or the absence of protest. It can also be deduced from specific circumstances as reasonably perceived by an ordinary individual.

Implied consent manifests when the prevailing circumstances reasonably suggest that consent has been granted, even without the direct articulation of agreement. Implied consent finds relevance in various situations where verbal or explicit consent is not expressly given but can be reasonably inferred based on actions, circumstances, or societal norms.

Here are instances where implied consent is applicable:

1. **Medical Procedures:** When a patient voluntarily presents themselves for routine medical check-ups or diagnostic tests, it is implied that they consent to standard procedures like measuring blood pressure, taking blood samples, or conducting physical examinations.In many countries, including the UAE, healthcare facilities that offer non-invasive procedures such as consultations are required to obtain General Consent from their patients, as stipulated by the country's laws. This is an important aspect of ensuring that patients are fully informed and aware of the treatments they will be receiving before providing their consent.

2. **Emergency Medical Care:** In situations where an individual is unconscious or unable to provide explicit consent due to a medical emergency, healthcare providers are often authorized to perform life-saving treatments based on the implied consent that the individual would want to be treated. Suppose a patient is unconscious and the legal Substitute Consent Giver is not available in non-emergency cases. In that case, the physician must consult with at least one other physician before providing treatment.

3. **Public Photography:** In public spaces, individuals often accept that their images may be captured by photographers or security cameras, implying their consent to be photographed or recorded for security or journalistic purposes.

4. **Website Cookies:** Many websites use cookies to collect user data. When users visit a website and continue to browse, they are often assumed to have given implied consent for the use of cookies as long as the website provides clear information and options for opting out.

5. **Childcare and Schools:** Parents implicitly consent to certain routine activities and safety measures when enrolling their children in schools or daycare centres, such as administering first aid or using photographs for school-related publications.

6. **Employment:** Employees may implicitly consent to specific workplace policies and practices, such as surveillance, security checks, and drug testing, when

accepting a job offer, provided these practices are legally disclosed.

7. **Social Etiquette:** In social interactions, implied consent plays a vital role. For example, when entering someone's home, it is generally assumed that you have implied consent to be a guest, and when shaking hands, there is implied consent for physical contact.

8. **Participation in Sports and Events:** Athletes and participants in sports and recreational events often consent to the inherent risks associated with the activity, implying consent to standard safety protocols and rules.

9. **Lending and Borrowing:** When people lend or borrow items among friends or acquaintances, there is often an implied understanding of the terms and conditions without the need for explicit agreements.

10. **Online Terms and Conditions:** When users accept or continue using online services, they may be seen as providing implied consent to the terms and conditions, including data collection and user agreements.

Implied consent, while not as explicit as verbal consent, is an essential concept that helps navigate various aspects of daily life and legal matters where clear, unspoken agreements guide our actions and expectations.

Implied consent primarily applies to routine and non-invasive medical procedures, like vital sign assessments or physical examinations. However, when dealing with more invasive, high-risk procedures, surgeries, or treatments, it becomes imperative to obtain explicit informed consent from the patient. This ensures that they fully understand the potential risks and benefits associated with these interventions and can make a well-informed decision about their medical care.

Patient Understanding is a pivotal aspect of implied consent in the healthcare context. This principle hinges on the premise that patients possess a comprehensive understanding of the healthcare procedures they are undergoing. However, it is imperative to note that when a patient is incapable of comprehending the nature of these procedures due to factors like mental incapacitation, implied consent may lose its validity. In such cases, healthcare providers must resort to alternative legal mechanisms, such as obtaining consent from a legal guardian, to ensure that the patient's rights are safeguarded.

Cultural and Ethical Considerations play a crucial role in shaping the boundaries of implied consent. It is essential to recognize that the definition of acceptable implied consent can exhibit variance across different cultures and belief systems. Therefore, healthcare professionals should exercise sensitivity towards these diversities and seek explicit consent when the need arises.

Nonetheless, it is important to acknowledge the Legal Risks associated with implied consent. Misinterpretation of a patient's actions or a failure to obtain explicit consent, when mandated, may render healthcare providers liable for medical malpractice or battery, making legal repercussions a genuine concern.

State and Institutional Regulations further compound the complexity of implied consent. Healthcare laws and regulations fluctuate between jurisdictions, and individual healthcare institutions often possess their distinct policies regarding consent.

Therefore, it is of utmost importance that healthcare professionals remain well-informed about local laws and institutional guidelines to ensure strict compliance.

3.2 Verbal Consent

Verbal consent, also known as Informed Consent with Waiver of Documentation, is the act of a patient expressing their consent for a medical procedure verbally, without the need for a written form. This practice is deemed sufficient for routine medical treatments such as diagnostic procedures and prophylaxis, provided comprehensive records are meticulously maintained. In this process, the investigator must adhere to the exact stringent requirements as with written consent, but in this case, the subject abstains from physically signing a consent form. It is crucial to note that a waiver of documentation of consent is only permissible under specific, limited circumstances. One fundamental prerequisite for such a waiver is that the research involved should not exceed a minimal risk threshold. This practice is often colloquially referred to as "verbal consent."

Verbal consent suits specific scenarios such as emergency medical procedures, routine diagnostic tests, and simple preventive treatments. Nonetheless, it is essential to guarantee that the patient has a complete understanding of the procedure's nature, potential risks, and available alternatives before proceeding with verbal consent. To ensure ethical and legal compliance, rigorous adherence to best practices for obtaining and documenting verbal consent is mandatory. Foremost, the healthcare provider must engage in transparent and comprehensive communication with the patient, elucidating the procedure, its purpose, potential risks, and addressing any questions or concerns in plain language, avoiding medical jargon. Once the patient has given their verbal consent, it should be meticulously recorded in the patient's medical records, specifying the date, time, and the healthcare professional's name who obtained the consent. Furthermore, it is advisable to have a witness present during this process to validate the patient's agreement. In critical situations where obtaining written consent is impractical, verbal consent becomes pivotal in ensuring prompt medical care while upholding patients' rights and ethical principles. Healthcare providers must prioritize clarity, transparency, and accurate documentation when utilizing this approach.

When it comes to verbal consents, a state of confusion may arise, where the information may not be delivered correctly, or the patient might not have understood it completely. This leaves loose ends and may create a conflict in the future. Thus, it is highly advisable that a written content system follows a verbal constent.

3.3 Written Consent

Written consent, in essence, is the formal act of granting permission for medical treatment. It entails the explicit agreement, expressed by a patient's signature on a consent form, to undergo specific medical procedures or therapies. This signed document assumes foremost importance in the medical domain, as it serves as a legally binding authorization that empowers healthcare professionals to proceed with the proposed treatment plan. By providing written consent, patients affirm their understanding and approval of the recommended interventions, contributing to transparency and accountability in the medical decision-making process. This practice not only safeguards the patient's rights but also ensures a comprehensive and ethical healthcare experience.

Written Consent includes a clear and concise description of the proposed medical procedure or treatment, ensuring that patients fully comprehend the nature of the intervention. Additionally, it outlines the potential risks, benefits, and alternatives, enabling patients to make informed choices. The consent form also encompasses a section detailing the credentials and qualifications of the healthcare provider performing the procedure, bolstering trust. Importantly, it must stipulate that consent is voluntary and can be withdrawn at any time. Furthermore, it should specify whether the procedure may involve any experimental aspects or research implications. Finally, the form must provide space for the patient's signature, signifying their understanding and willingness to proceed, culminating in a legally binding document that upholds ethical and legal standards.

1. **Engaging in Clinical Trials:** When patients decide to partake in a clinical trial, they are furnished with an informed consent document. This comprehensive document encapsulates vital information concerning the trial's objectives, procedural aspects, potential risks, and expected advantages. To actively engage in the trial, participants are obligated to meticulously review and affix their signature on the document, signifying their voluntary involvement and comprehensive understanding of the intricacies of the trial.

2. **Voluntary Blood Donation:** In the noble act of blood donation, individuals are presented with a written consent form that delineates the donation process, safety

protocols, and potential side effects. Donors are required to peruse and formally endorse this consent form, thereby acknowledging their wholehearted willingness to contribute their blood. This written consent plays a pivotal role in ensuring that donors possess a lucid comprehension of the donation process and are enthusiastic contributors.

3. **Facilitating Organ Donation:** For individuals who harbor the desire to be organ donors, expressing consent in writing can be achieved through an organ donation card or the act of registering as an organ donor on their driver's license. This written consent serves as an unambiguous declaration of the individual's intent to posthumously donate their organs, granting healthcare providers the authority to honor their heartfelt wishes, ultimately contributing to the noble cause of organ donation.

4. **Blood Transfusion:** In cases where a patient requires a blood transfusion, a healthcare provider discusses the need for this procedure, its potential benefits, and risks. The patient or their legal guardian is asked if they consent to the blood transfusion, and their verbal agreement is obtained. This ensures that the patient or their guardian is aware of the treatment and agrees to it.

5. Any surgical procedure involving incision of skin or mucosa: In these cases, the patient must be informed of the healing process and the several risks it holds, such as allergic reactions, scars or even grave skin conditions such as keliods.

6. Any invasive diagnostic procedure: When it comes to invasive diagnostic procedures, such as colonoscopy or

even a small biopsy, the patient can be exposed to health hazards, such as various cross infections.

7. Pre-op Assessment: Pre-op assessment plays a vital role in making the operation a smooth and hassle free process. The patient however, must be informed of the basic requirements such as hygiene maintenance, shaving, diet protocols, etc.

8. Surgical or invasive procedures: Surgical or invasive producers can have several health hazards, such as cross infection, delay in healing, hemorrhage, or even death. The patient must be asked to sign a content form which clearly lists out all the possible hazards of the procedure.

9. Any form of Anaesthesia: There are three main types of anaesthesia: topical, local, and general. Each of these procedures has its own hazards. For instance, the patient might be allergic to lidocaine or procaine used in topical anaesthesia and develop an allergic reaction to it. The patient must be informed of these possible hazards beforehand.

10. Chemotherapy and radiation therapy: These therapies have several hazards associated with them, such as alopecia or hair loss, sudden weight loss, fatigue, etc. The patient must be informed of these possibilities and a written consent must be signed.

3.4 Digital Consent

Digital consent, often referred to as e-consent, encompasses the electronic methods such as electronic health records, mobile apps, or telemedicine platforms, employed to obtain permission for various purposes, including healthcare interventions. In an increasingly digital age, digital consent has gained remarkable significance. It involves the use of electronic platforms and secure technologies to obtain a patient's informed approval for medical treatments, procedures, or data sharing. This method, while expedient and accessible, necessitates a nuanced examination of its advantages and challenges. The advantages of digital consent are evident in its efficiency, convenience, and the potential to streamline administrative processes within healthcare institutions. Patients can provide consent remotely, reducing the need for physical paperwork and in-person visits, which is particularly beneficial in telemedicine and during the COVID-19 pandemic. Moreover, digital consent allows for easier documentation and retrieval of consent records, enhancing accountability and transparency in healthcare.

However, digital consent also poses certain challenges, notably concerning security and privacy. The risk of data breaches and unauthorized access to sensitive medical information is a critical concern. Healthcare providers must implement robust encryption and cybersecurity measures to safeguard patient data. Furthermore, ensuring that patients fully understand the digital consent process and the implications of their consent remains a challenge. In healthcare, legal considerations are paramount, as they dictate the validity of digital consent. Compliance with relevant laws, such as the Health Insurance Portability and Accountability Act (HIPAA) in the United States, is essential to ensure that patient rights are protected. In conclusion, digital consent offers numerous advantages in healthcare, but it necessitates a comprehensive approach to security, privacy, and legal compliance to maintain its integrity and trustworthiness in an evolving digital landscape.

1. **Telemedicine Consultation:** In the domain of telemedicine, patients provide formal digital consent to partake in virtual medical consultations with their healthcare providers. This explicit agreement signifies their acknowledgment of using video conferencing or secure messaging platforms for diagnoses, treatment, or follow-up appointments. By consenting, both parties demonstrate their awareness of the remote nature of the consultation, as well as the potential associated risks and benefits.

2. **Health Data Research:** In the context of health data research, patients may formally grant digital consent for the utilization of their anonymized health data in medical studies. This formal consent grants healthcare institutions and researchers access to aggregated patient data while safeguarding individual privacy. It's imperative to highlight that patients retain the autonomy to participate or opt-out, which significantly contributes to scientific progress.

3. **Wearable Health Monitoring:** Wearable health monitoring is an area where patients formally provide digital consent for continuous health tracking. This consent permits the continuous collection of real-time data concerning vital signs, activity levels, and other essential health metrics. This formal agreement is crucial in ensuring patient autonomy and privacy when using digital tools to monitor and manage their health.

4. **Genetic Testing:** Patients can formally consent to genetic testing through digital platforms, granting permission to understand their genetic predispositions to specific health conditions. This digital consent ensures patients are well-

informed about the testing process, potential implications, and who will have access to their genetic information. Ultimately, it empowers patients to make well-considered decisions regarding genetic testing.

5. **Mobile Health Apps:** Patients frequently utilize mobile health apps for diverse healthcare purposes, including managing chronic conditions and monitoring medication adherence. Digital consent, a requisite formality, encompasses data sharing, privacy policies, and potential data utilization by app developers. It's imperative for patients to formally agree to these terms before engaging with the application.

In essence, medical treatment requires one's explicit consent unless it's a life-threatening emergency when one is unable to provide consent. Nevertheless, Patients and thier families possess the autonomy to decline treatment and information. In advance, you can designate a surrogate decision-maker through an advance directive or a legally binding document. Alternatively, you may opt for minimal information and entrust your healthcare provider with decision-making. It is important to note that informed consent laws mandate healthcare providers to share diagnoses with patients, even when requested by family members. Your right to make informed choices regarding your medical care is legally protected.

<u>CHAPTER 4: INFORMED CONSENT</u>

"Informed consent" is a fundamental process in which a patient acquires comprehensive knowledge about the purpose, advantages, and potential risks associated with medical procedures, including clinical research trials. Subsequently, the patient voluntarily agrees to undergo the treatment or participate in the trial. This practice is deeply rooted in ethical principles safeguarding rudimentary human rights and a legal framework.

Crucially, the patient holds the autonomy to make informed decisions regarding their body and gather pertinent information before undergoing any medical interventions. No individual, not even a physician, can compel the patient to follow a particular course of action. In this context, physicians serve as facilitators in the patient's decision-making process.

It is imperative to emphasize that obtaining informed consent is more than just a one-size-fits-all process achieved through a standardized consent form. Instead, it necessitates a case-specific approach tailored to the proposed procedure or treatment regimen. Despite the diligent practice of informed consent, neither medical practitioners nor healthcare facilities can absolve themselves from potential legal liabilities. Nevertheless, the patient is bound by the consent agreement, and deviation from the treatment specified in the signed informed consent can lead to a patient's dismissal by their physician.

4.1 Legal and Ethical Frameworks for Informed Consent

Legal Perspective:

An "informed consent" document, when signed by a patient, serves as a legal affirmation that the patient is willingly granting permission for a specific medical procedure at a designated time. From a legal perspective, it is essential to recognize that no one has the authority to touch, let alone treat, another individual without their explicit consent. This transgression can be legally classified as "battery," tantamount to physical assault, and is subject to legal repercussions. Consequently, obtaining informed consent is necessary for any medical procedure beyond a routine physical examination. The sole exception to this rule arises in medical emergencies, where a doctor may need to perform an operation without obtaining formal consent to save the patient's life. In such instances, the patient's survival is not guaranteed. Nevertheless, as long as the doctor acts competently, with due care and diligence, and in the best interests of the patient, they will not be held responsible for the patient's demise. To ensure valid informed consent, patients must be allowed to ask questions and seek clarifications, all without any form of coercion. Consent must be entirely voluntary, and the patient should retain the freedom to revoke it. If consent is given under duress, intimidation, or due to misconceptions or misrepresentation of facts, it may be deemed invalid.

Determining the validity of consent is a complex task akin to the validation of any contract. Irrespective of how meticulously a contract is crafted, its true validity is only confirmed when it undergoes scrutiny within a court of law. An illustrative case is that of Moore v. Regents of the University of California in July

1990, a landmark decision by the California Supreme Court. In this case, a patient who had signed an informed consent discovered that his blood cells possessed a unique property of stimulating the growth of white blood cells. Subsequently, these cells were utilized and patented, leading to financial gains for his doctor and the university. The court ultimately ruled that the patient, Moore, had no proprietary rights over his discarded cells or any profits derived from them. Nevertheless, it did find that the research physician had failed to disclose his financial interests in using Moore's cells. The court's consideration then extended to the overarching policy related to categorizing Moore's cells as property. The court expressed concern that granting property rights to tissues or organs would negatively impact medical research, given that exchanges involving property are subject to strict liability tort. Laboratories conducting research frequently receive substantial volumes of medical samples and cannot reasonably be expected to ascertain whether the origin of these samples was obtained illegally. As a result, Moore could only sue his doctor for the lack of disclosure, with no recourse against others. The case of Moore vividly underscores the potential pitfalls associated with informed consent for all parties involved.

"Informed consent" signifies a patient's voluntary agreement to undergo a specific medical procedure at a particular time. This consent is indispensable from a legal standpoint, as it safeguards individuals from unwanted physical intrusion and serves as the bedrock of medical ethics. Exceptions are limited to situations of medical emergency, where the necessity for immediate intervention overrides the requirement for formal consent. To ensure the validity of consent, patients must have the liberty to seek clarification, make informed choices, and withdraw their consent at any point. It is only through the scrutiny of the legal system that the true validity and consequences of informed consent become apparent, as exemplified by the case of Moore v. Regents of the University of California. This case highlights the intricate balance between patients' rights and the advancement of medical research, emphasizing the need for clear and transparent disclosure in the informed consent process.

Ethical Perspective:

A patient's assessment of the potential risks and advantages associated with a medical procedure is a highly individual, variable, and often unpredictable matter. In this context, it is crucial to ensure that patients receive comprehensive information that encompasses all pertinent risks. However, striving for an exhaustive catalog of potential risks and side effects is neither pragmatic nor feasible. To illustrate, most patients would find it daunting to comprehend the extensive product information leaflet accompanying a medication package. The informed consent documentation must be clearly legible, without any abbreviations, and completely free from medical jargon. What we should reasonably anticipate is that healthcare providers furnish patients with information that a rational individual can comprehend, enabling them to make informed decisions regarding their treatment options. It is imperative that patients have the opportunity to seek clarification and raise queries without any undue influence or pressure.

The question arises as to whether obtaining informed consent is, indeed, a necessary step. Some might contend that maintaining a solid doctor-patient relationship often proves more effective than relying solely on formal consent. Nevertheless, it remains pertinent to ponder the true value of "informed consent" if its validity can only be established through legal means. Furthermore, we must examine whether the concept of "informed consent" is rooted in legal mandates or ethical principles. If its origins lie primarily in the realm of legality, it may suggest that ethical considerations play a secondary role. However, it is essential to acknowledge that even if a practice is legally sound, it may not necessarily align with ethical standards, thus underscoring the significance of ethical dimensions within this context.

4.2 Components of Informed Consent Process

The multifaceted process of informed consent encompasses several vital components, all of which are integral for its effective execution. At its core, this process revolves around three fundamental elements: information disclosure and comprehension, voluntariness and the preservation of patient autonomy, and competence and decision-making capacity. By delving into these crucial facets, we can develop a comprehensive insight into how healthcare providers carefully manage the intricate equilibrium between upholding patients' rights and providing the highest standard of care. This complex interplay among these key elements is of paramount importance, as it ensures that patients are adequately informed, willingly participate, and possess the necessary capability to make well-informed decisions regarding their medical treatment, thereby fostering a harmonious partnership between healthcare providers and their patients.

(i) Information Disclosure and Comprehension

This integral aspect entails the ethical responsibility of healthcare practitioners to divulge pertinent information concerning the proposed treatment, which encompasses its purpose, potential risks, advantages, available alternatives, and the possible repercussions of declining the treatment.

- Purpose and Nature of Treatment: Healthcare providers are obligated to elucidate the essence and meaning of the treatment in a clear and intelligible manner. This entails delineating the intended outcomes, the treatment's objectives, and its alignment with the patient's comprehensive healthcare strategy.

- Risks and Benefits: Patients must be apprised of the conceivable dangers and benefits associated with the proposed treatment. This disclosure should encompass both common and rare complications, as well as potential side effects, allowing patients to make a discerning assessment of whether the anticipated benefits outweigh the accompanying risks.

- Alternative Treatments: Patients should be duly informed about any available alternative treatment options, together with their associated risks and benefits. This empowers patients to explore other avenues and make judicious choices in accordance with their personal preferences and values.

- Consequences of Refusal: The healthcare provider is charged with the responsibility of communicating the probable consequences of declining the recommended treatment, ensuring that patients comprehend the potential impact on their health. This enables patients to deliberate on the implications of non-adherence to the prescribed course of action.

(ii) Patient Autonomy and the Importance of Informed Consent

This underscores the significance of upholding patient autonomy, wherein individuals possess the inherent right to accept or decline medical interventions, uninhibited by external pressures.

- The Eradication of Coercion: Patients should never encounter coercion or feel pressured into making specific choices regarding their medical care. Healthcare providers have the ethical responsibility to foster an environment characterized by safety and impartiality, facilitating patients' free expression of their medical preferences.

- The Right to Refuse: In the realm of patient autonomy, individuals hold the right to reject any medical intervention, even if it contradicts the recommendation of their healthcare provider. This autonomy extends to decisions concerning the continuation or cessation of treatment.

- Comprehensive Understanding of Options: Crucial to patient autonomy is the necessity for patients to possess a lucid comprehension of the alternatives and ramifications associated with their decisions. This knowledge ensures that their choices are well-informed and align with their values and personal preferences.

- Assessment of Decision-Making Capacity: The healthcare provider's role extends to evaluating a patient's decision-making capacity, encompassing their ability to comprehend the pertinent information, weigh the pros and cons, and communicate their choice effectively. In situations where a patient's capacity is compromised, additional support, such as the involvement of a surrogate decision-maker, may be required.

(iii) Competence and Decision-Making Capacity in Informed Consent

The assessment of competence and decision-making capacity is pivotal in the informed consent procedure within healthcare. It is incumbent upon healthcare providers to thoroughly appraise a patient's ability to comprehend and deliberate on their medical choices. This becomes particularly pertinent in scenarios where patients grapple with cognitive impairments or mental health issues.

- Capacity Evaluation: The crucial determination of whether the patient possesses the requisite decision-making capacity. This assessment encompasses a comprehensive evaluation of the patient's ability to grasp, appreciate, employ reason, and effectively convey their choices concerning the proposed medical interventions.

- Cognitive Impairments: Patients contending with cognitive impairments, such as dementia, may exhibit fluctuations in their decision-making capacity. In such instances, healthcare professionals must delve into a nuanced analysis of whether the patient possesses "decision-specific capacity" - the capability to render decisions concerning a particular treatment, even in instances where they may lack general decision-making capacity.

- **Surrogate Decision-Makers:** In those unfortunate situations where patients lack the capacity to make decisions autonomously, surrogate decision-makers, often comprising family members or legally appointed guardians, may need to intervene on the patient's behalf. The selection of these surrogates should be a meticulously conducted process, ensuring that the chosen individuals are well-versed in the patient's values and preferences. This ensures that decisions made align with the patient's best interests.

4.4 Challenges and Issues in Obtaining Informed Consent in Healthcare

Obtaining informed consent in the complex and diverse healthcare landscape can be a multifaceted effort fraught with challenges. Owing to cultural and linguistic obstacles, decision-making during emergencies and critical situations, and the unique challenges of obtaining consent from vulnerable populations.

Cultural diversity is a defining hallmark of contemporary healthcare. Patients hailing from various cultural backgrounds bring with them a rich tapestry of belief systems, traditions, and languages. These elements often pose significant impediments to the acquisition of informed consent.

Language disparities, a frequent occurrence in healthcare settings, present a formidable challenge. Patients who do not share a common language with their healthcare provider may struggle to comprehend the information presented, thereby hindering their capacity to provide genuine informed consent. In response, healthcare facilities frequently rely on interpreters and translation services to bridge this linguistic gap. Nevertheless, effective communication goes beyond mere translation; it must encompass the nuances and sensitivities of different cultures.

Cultural diversity also introduces variations in how patients perceive illness, treatment, and the concept of informed consent itself. Certain cultures may place great emphasis on communal decision-making, where the patient's family assumes a central role in the consent process. In contrast, individualistic cultures prioritize the autonomy of the patient. Navigating these cultural disparities requires sensitivity and respect for the patient's unique wishes and values.

To address these formidable cultural and linguistic barriers, healthcare institutions must invest in interpreter services, culturally competent training for their staff, and comprehensive patient education materials available in multiple languages. Furthermore, healthcare providers must demonstrate adaptability by tailoring informed consent discussions to align with the patient's specific cultural context.

In healthcare, certain situations do not afford the luxury of time for in-depth discussions about informed consent. Emergencies and critical conditions frequently necessitate swift decision-making to preserve a patient's life. This presents a complex ethical quandary, where the imperative of acquiring approval must be balanced with the exigency of delivering timely care.

Implied Consent emerges as a pivotal concept in numerous emergency scenarios wherein a patient cannot provide explicit consent due to their condition. It operates under the premise that a reasonable person would grant approval for essential treatment if they could do so. Nevertheless, ascertaining what precisely constitutes "essential treatment" can provoke disputes.

Decision-Making in Emergencies and Critical Conditions:

Proxy Decision-Makers are indispensable when patients are incapacitated, rendering them incapable of decision-making. These decision-makers, typically family members or legal guardians, may need to be responsible for granting consent on the patient's behalf. This process can be intricate, mainly when complicated family dynamics come into play or when there is no designated decision-maker. The perpetual challenge lies in striking a delicate balance between the imperative for expeditious medical intervention and the ethical obligation of informed consent. Healthcare providers are mandated to adhere to established protocols and guidelines, and in cases of uncertainty, they may involve ethics committees to ensure judicious decision-making under the duress of high-pressure situations.

Vulnerable Populations and Consent Challenges:

Vulnerable populations, comprising children, the elderly, individuals with limited cognitive capacity, and those mentally incapacitated, require particular consideration when seeking informed consent—the complexities in obtaining such consent stem from the unique characteristics of these groups.

Firstly, minors lack the legal capacity to grant informed consent independently. Instead, medical decisions on their behalf are typically made by parents or legal guardians. Nonetheless, recognizing the evolving maturity of children, it is imperative to respect their increasing ability to participate in decision-making.

Hence, the provision of age-appropriate information becomes paramount.

Secondly, elderly patients often grapple with cognitive decline, rendering it difficult for them to comprehend the consequences of medical decisions fully. Healthcare providers must conduct individual capacity assessments and, where necessary, engage family members or legal representatives.

Furthermore, patients suffering from mental illnesses, particularly severe dementia, may not possess the mental capacity to provide informed consent. In such cases, surrogate decision-makers are commonly involved, but ethical dilemmas concerning the patient's best interests may arise. Addressing the consent challenges inherent to these vulnerable populations necessitates the establishment of clear guidelines and policies within healthcare settings. Furthermore, involving ethics committees, legal experts, and family members in the decision-making process is essential to ensure that the best interests of the patient are upheld. This multifaceted approach aims to navigate the intricate ethical terrain surrounding informed consent for these groups.

Vulnerable populations present distinctive challenges when seeking informed consent, demanding a nuanced approach that respects the evolving capacities of children, addresses cognitive decline in the elderly, and deals with ethical concerns related to mentally incapacitated individuals. Establishing robust guidelines and involving relevant stakeholders in the decision-making process are integral components.

4.4. Improving the Informed Consent Process

It revolves around a patient's voluntary concurrence to undergo medical treatment, grounded in a comprehensive grasp of the concomitant risks, benefits, and available alternatives. Effective informed consent is paramount in upholding patient autonomy and fostering ethical healthcare practices. This exposition delves into how healthcare professionals can enhance the informed consent process via proficient communication methodologies, embracing shared decision-making with a patient-centric approach, and harnessing technology to augment procedural aspects.

Patients ought to receive information in a lucid, comprehensible manner, free from obfuscating jargon or intricate medical terminology. Healthcare providers are thus tasked with deploying several communication strategies to fulfill this:

- Plain Language: The employment of simple and unadorned language when elucidating medical procedures, potential risks, and associated benefits is pivotal. This practice circumvents potential linguistic barriers, thereby ensuring that patients can fully apprehend the disseminated information.

- Visual Aids: The integration of visual aids, encompassing diagrams, videos, and infographics, is pivotal in facilitating comprehension. Such tools distill intricate medical concepts, rendering the information more accessible and intelligible for patients.

- Teach-Back Method: Post information provision, healthcare practitioners may invite patients to 'teach back' what they have imbibed. This technique not only validates comprehension but also pinpoints areas necessitating further elucidation.

- Timing: Deliberations pertaining to informed consent should remain unhurried. Healthcare providers are well-advised to allocate ample time for addressing patient queries and concerns. This, in turn, mitigates the prospect of patients feeling unduly pressured, ensuring they make decisions in a reflective and considerate manner.

In essence, the crux of enhancing the informed consent process hinges on effective communication strategies that promote comprehension, reinforce patient autonomy, and uphold the ethical underpinnings of healthcare provision. Such efforts serve as a testament to the dedication of healthcare professionals to the welfare of their patients and the principles of ethical medical practice

4.5 Types of Informed Consents

1. General Informed Consent

A general informed consent form is an understanding between a patient and their healthcare provider. It includes:

- This consent allows the doctor to do routine consultations and physical examinations. It also includes non-invasive diagnostic tests like blood pressure checks or X-rays.
- It discusses the permissions for the doctor has to discuss a patient's case with other doctors and hospital staff.
- The document also discusses a patient's right to ask questions, obtain medical records, and refuse treatment or tests.

- Patients' responsibilities would also be listed, which would include need to provide accurate information about their health history.

2. Procedure-Specific Consent

Procedure-specific informed consent forms provide detailed information about a particular medical procedure. They include:

- All the specific details about the procedure must be included in this consent form. This also includes the risks and side effects the procedure might have.
- Next, it must also include all the alternate treatment options the patient would have. This must also include their procedures, risks and side effects respectively. This shall help the patient to make an informed decision.
- Furthermore, the form also talks about the recovery process. It enlists all the management strategies and the post-operative care that might be necessary.
- If anesthesia is involved, the form will explain the type used and potential risks.

3. Transfer Consent

A transfer consent form is necessary when patients are being shifted from one place to another. This can be from one hospital to another or to any other destination. It may also include an ambulance transfer or a transfer of a doctor. These forms talk about:

- The document will outline the reason for the transfer and the receiving facility's capabilities.
- It confirms the patient's consent to share his/her/their medical information with the receiving facility to ensure continuity of care.

- The form may briefly outline the potential risks and benefits associated with the transfer, such as potential delays or discomfort.
- It can also explain the cost implications associated with transfer and any additional provisions of care related to it.

Benefits: Transfer consent ensures a smooth transition of care between healthcare providers and facilities.

4. Admission Consent

Admission consent forms are obtained every time patients are admitted to a hospital for treatment. They typically cover:

- The form may outline any specific procedures planned during patients stay, such as surgery or diagnostic tests.
- It may explain the hospital's policies regarding medication administration, visitors, and costs related to admission and discharge procedures.
- The form may briefly outline patients expected financial obligations for the hospital stay.

Benefits: Admission consent clarifies the patient's agreement to the terms of hospital stay and ensures everyone is on the same page.

5. Refusal Consents

Refusal consent empowers patients to decline any recommended treatment or procedure. These come in various forms:

- Refusal for Treatment/Procedure Consent: This document allows patients to formally refuse a specific treatment or procedure. It is crucial to understand that refusing recommended treatment may have consequences, and the form may require patients to acknowledge these risks.

- Leave Against Medical Advice (LAMA): A LAMA form documents patients decision to leave the hospital against their doctor's recommendation. It typically requires patients to acknowledge the potential risks associated with leaving early or without seeking recommended treatment or procedure.

- Discharge Against Medical Advice (DAMA): Similar to a LAMA, a DAMA form documents patient's decision to leave the hospital before the doctor feels it is safe to do so. Hospitals may require a responsible adult to take legal responsibility for patient's care upon discharge.

- In cases where patients refuse to sign LAMA or DAMA, the organizations should be robust processes in place to validate such departures against medical advice through a organizational escalation or joint leadership decisions.

CHAPTER 5: CLINICAL SCENARIOS

5.1 Consent in Pediatric Care:

The process of obtaining informed consent for minors pertains to granting approval for medical procedures when the patient is under 18, not of legal adulthood. Although minors lack legal consent capacity like adults, their assent is often sought along with parental or guardian consent for their cooperation in care. This multifaceted decision-making involves assessing the minor's varying comprehension levels and involvement. Hence, obtaining consent In case of minors involves navigating a complex landscape where parental or guardian involvement plays a crucial role. This process acknowledges not only legal but also ethical and developmental factors in ensuring comprehensive healthcare decisions for minors.

Legal guardians or parents bear the fundamental responsibility of providing consent for minors, serving as primary decision-makers in pediatric care. They hold the authority to approve or refuse medical treatments or procedures, guided by the child's best interests, ensuring their health needs are met. Let's explore a few hypothetical clinical scenarios to gain a deeper insight into the intricacies of informed consent in pediatric care.

- Scenario 1: Vaccination of a 12-Year-Old Child: When a 12-year-old seeks routine vaccinations, the healthcare provider discusses the necessity and advantages of the procedure with both the child and their parents. Although legal decisions rest with the parents, the healthcare professional involves the child, ensuring their comprehension and seeking their agreement. This delicate balance upholds the child's autonomy while acknowledging the parental legal authority. This collaborative process underscores the importance of informed decision-making in pediatric care, where the minor's understanding and the guardians' consent align for the best possible healthcare outcomes. The "Gillick competence" is a widely recognized assessment of capability in the NHS, UK. It allows minors under the age of 16 to give their consent to their own treatment, provided they are deemed to possess sufficient intelligence, competence, and understanding to fully comprehend the implications of their treatment. This is known as being Gillick competent. In cases where the minor is not Gillick competent, their parent or legal guardian is authorized to provide consent on their behalf.

- Scenario 2: Emergency Medical Treatment for a Minor: Imagine a scenario where a 16-year-old is rushed to the emergency room after a severe accident. The medical team swiftly intervenes to stabilize the minor's condition. In emergency situations, the priority is to provide immediate medical care to preserve the minor's life or prevent additional harm. Once the situation stabilizes, the focus shifts towards engaging the parents or legal guardians to obtain informed consent for any necessary follow-up treatment or procedures. Consent can be sought before emergency care, but patient safety is always the top priority in an emergency. This situation underscores the crucial balance between the urgency of medical intervention and the significance of securing consent from guardians to ensure ongoing care aligns with the minor's best interests.

- Scenario 3: Adolescent Mental Health Treatment: When adolescents seek mental health treatment, they may encounter reluctance to involve their parents due to stigma or personal concerns. In these instances, the laws concerning minors' rights to consent to mental health services without parental involvement can differ based on the jurisdiction. Healthcare professionals are entrusted with delicately navigating these complex scenarios, ensuring the confidentiality of minors while upholding legal and ethical standards. In certain circumstances, these guidelines might allow minors to seek treatment without requiring parental consent, underscoring the elaborate balance between safeguarding a minor's autonomy and ensuring their well-being.

- Scenario 4: Adolescent Reproductive Health Confidentiality: In this scenario, a 15-year-old girl attends a reproductive health clinic seeking birth control. She expresses concerns about her parents' reaction and emphasizes the need for confidentiality. The healthcare provider encounters a complex situation, as legal and ethical norms in some regions might allow minors to consent to reproductive health services independently. The provider grapples with the moral balance between honouring the minor's right to confidentiality and considering the potential health risks without parental involvement. This dilemma poses a challenging ethical scenario frequently encountered by healthcare providers in adolescent care, navigating the delicate intersection of legal frameworks and the best interests of the young patient.

- Scenario 5: Chronic Illness Management in a Teen: When dealing with a 17-year-old diagnosed with a chronic illness seeking alternative treatments, a clash emerges between the minor's wish and the parents' firm belief in conventional medicine. The healthcare team encounters a delicate situation as the minor nears legal adulthood. Balancing the minor's autonomy in decision-making while prioritizing their well-being becomes complex, particularly if the alternative treatments contradict the parents' preferences and established medical practices. This intricacy arises due to the approaching legal age of the minor, necessitating a thoughtful consideration of both the minor's preferences and the medical necessity based on established practices.

- Scenario 6: Surgical Intervention for a Newborn: In an urgent scenario, a newborn with a congenital condition necessitates immediate surgical intervention. The parents, facing understandable apprehension, grapple with the potential risks associated with the procedure. The healthcare team plays a crucial role by furnishing detailed information about the surgery, emphasizing its urgency, and outlining possible outcomes. Despite this guidance, the ultimate decision rests with the parents, highlighting the delicate balance required between the best interest of the infant and the parent's capacity to grasp and make informed decisions for their child's well-being It is always recommended that physicians understand the local jurisdictions and regulatory framework they are practising in. At large such decisions are guided by legal and regulatory policies.

Navigating pediatric consent involves sophistication in ethical considerations. Balancing beneficence, non-maleficence, autonomy, and justice presents challenges, especially when a minor's decision conflicts with their guardians' perceived best interest. Legal frameworks and professional guidelines vary across regions, adding layers of complexity to the consent process. Understanding and navigating these nuances becomes crucial for safeguarding the well-being and rights of minors while respecting the roles of those responsible for their care. As the healthcare landscape evolves, the ongoing discourse on informed consent for minors remains an indispensable aspect of ethical healthcare practices, requiring continual adaptation and attention.

5.2 Consent in Mental Health Care

In cases involving individuals with mental health conditions, the ethical principles and legal standards governing informed consent take on intricate dimensions. In such situations, where the patient's decision-making capacity may be compromised, healthcare providers face challenging ethical dilemmas. Balancing the patient's autonomy and well-being becomes a delicate task, necessitating careful consideration of the individual's specific condition and the need to safeguard their rights while providing appropriate care.

Understanding Informed Consent in Mental Health - Decision-Making Challenges:

In mental health care, decision-making capacity stands as a crucial aspect. Conditions affecting mental health often hinder one's ability to fully grasp the nature, risks, and implications of proposed treatments. Consider someone in a manic episode due to bipolar disorder—altered judgment and perception may impair their capacity to make informed choices about treatment. It's a delicate balance—healthcare professionals must respect patients' autonomy while ensuring their well-being. Assessing an individual's capacity to decide requires a nuanced approach. For instance, a person with severe depression might still possess decision-making capacity, whereas someone in acute psychosis may lack it due to their altered mental state. Striking this balance between autonomy and care is vital in navigating the complexities of informed consent in mental health.

Guardianship and Consent in Psychiatric Treatment - Legal and Ethical Considerations

In situations where individuals cannot autonomously decide on psychiatric treatment, legal guardians or substitute decision-makers play a pivotal role. These designated individuals, often family members or court-appointed guardians, hold legal authority to make treatment decisions for those lacking decision-making capacity. However, laws governing guardianship can differ between regions. The ethical landscape in this scenario is complex. Guardians are responsible for acting in the best interests of the person they represent. This duty involves aligning decisions with the individual's known wishes, values, and overall well-being. Yet, challenges arise when the person's preferences are unclear or clash with the guardian's perception of what's best for the individual. Navigating these ethical quandaries forms a significant part of the guardian's role in psychiatric care.

Case Scenarios and Real-Life Examples

- Scenario 1: Schizophrenia and Informed Consent: Imagine a situation where an individual is diagnosed with schizophrenia. In the throes of acute psychosis, this person might lack the mental capacity necessary to comprehend and decide about their treatment. In such instances, healthcare providers might need to turn to legal guardians or designated decision-makers to ensure the person receives essential care and treatment.

- Scenario 2: Bipolar Disorder and Varied Capacity: In cases of bipolar disorder, the condition's fluctuating nature poses a challenge in evaluating decision-making capacity. During manic episodes, individuals might display impaired judgment, affecting their ability to provide informed consent for treatment. However, during stable periods, their capability to make decisions about their care might be different, showing a notable variance in their ability to understand and consent to treatment options.

- Scenario 3: Resisting Treatment in Severe Depression: Picture an individual diagnosed with severe depression who staunchly refuses treatment despite the gravity of their condition. Although competent in daily activities, they hold firm in the belief that no treatment will assuage their distress. This poses a predicament for the healthcare team: while respecting the person's decision is crucial, their refusal of treatment could endanger their well-being. This dilemma requires a careful balance between respecting the individual's autonomy and preventing potential harm from untreated severe depression.

- Scenario 4: Substance Use Disorder's Impact on Decision-Making: Imagine an individual contending with substance use disorder, where decision-making abilities fluctuate significantly during intoxication or withdrawal. Consent for treatment might be given while sober, but this capacity varies with their substance use patterns. Determining the appropriate moment for seeking informed consent becomes challenging due to the individual's changing mental state, affecting their ability to make consistent and rational decisions.

- Scenario 5: Intellectual Disability and Treatment Decision-Making: In cases involving individuals with intellectual disabilities, consistent limitations in decision-making capacity prevail. Understanding complex treatment options and their consequences might be beyond their grasp. Here, the challenge lies in acquiring consent and ensuring that proposed treatments align with the individual's best interests and ethical considerations. Legal guardians or family members take on a crucial role in making decisions that prioritize the person's welfare while upholding their autonomy as much as possible. These scenarios underscore the intricate balance between autonomy and well-being in the realm of informed consent.

Mitigating Challenges and Ensuring Ethical Practices

A crucial strategy in navigating the complexities of decision-making in mental health care involves a multidisciplinary approach. Healthcare teams integrate expertise from psychiatrists, psychologists, social workers, and legal professionals to holistically assess an individual's ability to make informed choices regarding their treatment. The collaborative evaluation considers various aspects such as cognitive abilities, emotional state, and understanding of the treatment process. Addressing these intricacies, advance directives stand as pivotal tools. These documents empower individuals to articulate their treatment preferences and appoint a trusted advocate who can aid in decision-making during periods of reduced capacity. Moreover, supported decision-making models enable individuals to make choices in tandem with trusted supporters, preserving as much autonomy as possible. This comprehensive approach respects a person's autonomy and ensures that their treatment preferences are valued, even in situations where their decision-making capacity might be compromised.

Balancing the rights of autonomy with the responsibility of care within the realm of mental health demands a nuanced approach. Employing a multidisciplinary assessment involving psychiatrists, psychologists, social workers, and legal professionals is crucial. Additionally, the utilization of advance directives permits individuals to outline treatment preferences and designate trusted decision-making support. This comprehensive approach enables healthcare providers to navigate the intricacies of mental health ethically, ensuring the well-being of individuals dealing with mental health conditions while respecting their autonomy.

5.3 Consent in Research and Experimental Treatments

In the continually evolving healthcare sector, research and experimental treatments are crucial drivers for advancing medical science, devising innovative therapies, and enhancing patient care. Nevertheless, these efforts are rooted in a fundamental ethical tenet: informed consent. This comprehensive article delves into the intricate landscape of informed consent, particularly focusing on its significance in clinical trials. It also examines the ethical complexities surrounding emergency scenarios and the potential for waived consent, shedding light on the intricate ethical aspects underpinning these medical practices.

Informed Consent in Clinical Trials and Research:

In medical research, clinical trials are a methodical and scientific means to assess the safety and effectiveness of novel therapies, medications, and medical procedures. At the core of these trials and research lies the pivotal component of informed consent, ensuring that individuals comprehend the research, its potential outcomes, and their involvement. The process of securing informed consent within clinical trials acts as a multifaceted safeguard, aiming to uphold the rights and welfare of those participating in the research. This intricate process involves several critical components:

The cornerstone of ethical clinical research, informed consent, is a multifaceted process designed to safeguard the rights and well-being of research participants. This comprehensive process includes providing potential participants with a clear and thorough understanding of the research, encompassing its purpose, procedures, potential risks, benefits, and alternatives. This information should be conveyed in a language and format that participants can readily comprehend.

Scenario: Let's consider a practical scenario where a pharmaceutical company conducts a clinical research to evaluate a novel drug for a rare medical condition. In this case, the informed consent document plays a pivotal role by meticulously detailing the medical condition in question, the investigational drug, its potential side effects, and the likelihood of benefits. This comprehensive disclosure empowers participants to make informed decisions about their involvement in the trial, ensuring that their autonomy and well-being are respected throughout the research process.

Voluntariness: Voluntariness is vital to the informed consent process during clinical research. Participants must freely and willingly choose to be part of the research without any undue influence, coercion, or unrealistic promises of benefits. They should always have the option to decline or withdraw from the study without facing negative consequences.

For instance, consider a scenario where a patient diagnosed with a life-threatening illness is approached to participate in a clinical trial. In this case, it is imperative to ensure that the patient's decision to participate is not driven by fear or pressure related to their illness but is a genuine and voluntary commitment to contribute to advancing medical science.

Capacity: It is a pivotal component of informed consent, necessitating that research participants possess the mental and emotional ability to comprehend information and make informed decisions. A legally authorized representative steps in to provide consent for individuals lacking this capacity.

Scenario: Consider scenarios involving vulnerable populations like individuals with severe cognitive impairments. In such cases, involving a legal guardian or family member in the consent process becomes crucial to safeguard the best interests of the participant. This ensures that decisions are aligned with their well-being and care.

Continual Dialogue: The informed consent process extends beyond a single interaction, fostering ongoing communication between researchers and participants throughout the study's duration. This continual exchange ensures that participants can express concerns, seek clarifications, and make informed choices regarding their involvement.

Scenario: In long-term clinical trials or research, participants might encounter unforeseen health changes or unexpected side effects. The ongoing dialogue enables participants to address these developments, empowering them to make well-informed decisions regarding their continued participation in the study.

The Ethical Importance of Informed Consent

Informed consent forms the ethical core of clinical trials, embodying crucial ethical principles:

- Transparency: It ensures full disclosure of information, such as the research's purpose, risks, benefits, and available alternatives, enabling participants to make informed decisions.

- Autonomy: Participants volunteer without coercion, maintaining the freedom to withdraw at any stage without repercussion.

- Respect: It honours an individual's right to self-determination and protects their well-being during research participation.

It also upholds several vital ethical principles in clinical trials:

a) Respecting Individual Autonomy: Informed consent is anchored in the crucial principle of recognizing and honouring an individual's right to self-determination in matters concerning their body and health.

Scenario: Consider a situation where a patient diagnosed with cancer is presented with the choice to join a clinical trial for a new chemotherapy approach or pursue standard treatment. Upholding the principle of autonomy, the patient should have the liberty to make a decision aligned with their personal values and preferences, ensuring their active involvement in the decision-making process.

b) Beneficence: It is a critical ethical principle in the context of informed consent that safeguards participants in clinical trials. Ensuring that research maximizes benefits and minimizes harm prevents participants from being exposed to unproven or risky treatments without their explicit awareness and consent.

For example, when conducting a clinical trial involving a novel medical device, it is imperative to prioritize participant well-being. This consists in providing comprehensive information about potential risks, closely monitoring their progress throughout the study, and adhering to rigorous safety protocols to uphold the principle of beneficence.

c) Non-Maleficence: Upholding the principle of non-maleficence means that researchers must avoid causing harm to research participants. Informed consent serves as a critical tool, empowering participants to thoroughly evaluate potential risks and make informed decisions regarding their involvement in the research.

Scenario: Consider a clinical trial focused on testing a new vaccine. It is imperative that the informed consent process provides a detailed account of potential side effects associated with the vaccine. This transparency allows participants to carefully assess the risks, including adverse reactions, in comparison to the potential benefits of immunization, thus ensuring their well-being remains prominent.

d) Justice: The ethical principle of justice underscores the importance of fairness and non-discrimination in research. Informed consent is pivotal in ensuring that research participants are chosen impartially and that vulnerable populations are not exploited. It promotes equal access to research opportunities, reducing the likelihood of undue bias in participant selection.

Scenario: In the recruitment process for a clinical trial, researchers must adhere to objective criteria when selecting participants, avoiding any influence from socioeconomic or demographic factors that could lead to biased or unfair recruitment practices.

Informed Consent in Clinical Research Practice

Let's delve into specific scenarios to better understand informed consent within clinical trials.

Scenario 1: A Phase III Clinical Trial for a New Cancer Drug

The comprehensive informed consent process is fundamental in a Phase III clinical trial conducted by a pharmaceutical company to assess a new cancer drug. It initiates during the recruitment phase, where potential participants receive extensive information about the trial's goals, the experimental drug, and the potential risks and benefits. This transparent communication is pivotal in ensuring their understanding and decision-making process.

Throughout the trial's duration, participants maintain regular contact with the research team, fostering health monitoring and continual data collection. Any new insights into the drug's safety or effectiveness are promptly relayed to the participants, encouraging an open channel for questions and clarification.

Upon the trial's completion, participants are briefed about the findings and their vital contribution to advancing cancer treatment. They are granted the choice to continue receiving the drug if it proves efficacious or revert to standard therapy. This emphasis on participant autonomy and well-being is a consistent priority throughout the trial process, ensuring their involvement is informed and respected.

Scenario 2: Informed Consent in Pediatric Clinical Trials

Special attention to informed consent is vital in clinical trials involving children. Typically, parents or legal guardians grant consent on the child's behalf. However, as children mature, their assent may also be sought to participate in the research.

For instance, in a pediatric clinical trial evaluating a new vaccine, parents receive comprehensive details about the trial, including potential benefits and risks, aiding them in making an informed decision for their child. As the child grows, the research team engages in age-appropriate discussions to ensure their understanding of the trial and comfort with participation. If capable of comprehending the research, their assent is requested.

In both contexts, informed consent stands as a crucial ethical aspect, ensuring respect for sovereignty and safeguarding the rights of research participants.

Emergency Situations and Waived Consent

In emergency medical situations, the paramount objective is to safeguard the patient's life or prevent substantial harm, prioritizing the ethical principle of beneficence. Healthcare providers may need to make swift decisions and initiate necessary treatments without the opportunity to secure formal consent. However, this scenario calls for a delicate balance between ensuring the patient's well-being and respecting their autonomy.

One solution to this ethical dilemma is waived or deferred consent. In such situations, where immediate action is imperative, healthcare providers may proceed with necessary treatments while making every effort to involve the patient or their surrogate decision-maker in the decision-making process as soon as practicable. This approach aims to uphold the patient's rights while acknowledging the practical constraints of emergency care.

Waived consent is typically allowed under strict legal and ethical guidelines, and it is essential to document the circumstances surrounding its application. Additionally, the patient's condition, response to treatment, and any subsequent decisions made once they regain capacity should be meticulously recorded to ensure transparency and accountability.

In summary, while informed consent is a fundamental ethical principle in healthcare, emergencies present unique challenges where immediate medical intervention is necessary. Waived consent, when used judiciously and in accordance with established guidelines, strikes a balance between beneficence and autonomy, ultimately serving the patient's best interests.

CHAPTER 6: WHO CAN GIVE CONSENT

6.1 Patient's Competent Consent

In healthcare decision-making, the authority to consent to a patient's care is assigned to different individuals, contingent on the situation. These key decision-makers include:

a) The Patient Themselves (If Competent)

The foundation of consent hinges on the patient's capacity to make well-informed choices regarding their health. Competent patients possess the legal and ethical authority to grant consent for their medical treatment. Competency is ascertained by the patient's ability to comprehend essential information related to their medical condition, available treatment options, associated risks, and potential benefits, enabling them to make rational decisions based on this understanding. In most regions, the law dictates the definition of "competent individual".

For instance, envision a scenario in which a patient receives a chronic illness diagnosis and is presented with multiple treatment options. In such a case, a competent patient, after receiving comprehensive information from healthcare professionals, can carefully evaluate the advantages and disadvantages of each treatment and make an informed decision aligned with their preferences and level of comprehension. This ensures that patient autonomy remains at the forefront of the decision-making process.

b) Legal Guardians or Representatives

When a patient lacks the capacity to provide consent, such as due to severe cognitive impairment or being a minor, the responsibility of decision-making falls on legal guardians or appointed representatives. These individuals obtain authority through court orders or legally binding documents, enabling them to act in the patient's best interest.

For instance, an individual experiencing advanced dementia might not comprehend medical treatments. In this scenario, a court-appointed legal guardian, often a family member or appointed representative, assumes the role of decision-maker, ensuring decisions align with the patient's best interests.

c) Healthcare Proxies: Also termed as Medical Power of Attorney, are appointed individuals chosen by competent patients to make medical decisions on their behalf in the event of their incapacity. This legal designation empowers the proxy to act in accordance with the patient's expressed wishes.

In a scenario where a patient is fully competent, they might create a healthcare proxy document designating a close friend to make healthcare decisions if the patient becomes incapacitated due to unforeseen circumstances, such as being in a coma following an accident.

d) Next of Kin: In healthcare decision-making, when a patient's preferences or legal documents aren't accessible, the next of kin, typically family members, are often involved in decision-making. However, their authority can vary based on legal and ethical considerations, especially if there are conflicting family opinions or unknown patient wishes.

In a scenario where an unconscious patient arrives at a hospital without identifiable documentation or an appointed representative, healthcare providers might turn to the patient's next of kin for decisions about treatment options.

e) Competence: In healthcare, decision-making relies on a patient's capacity to grasp relevant information, process it effectively, and articulate their preferences. This involves cognitive abilities, understanding, and the ability to make reasoned decisions. Assessing competence consists of evaluating a patient's grasp of their medical condition, the treatment, and its associated risks and benefits.

For instance, a patient facing a complex medical diagnosis receives thorough information about available treatments and their potential outcomes. The patient demonstrates a comprehensive understanding and articulates a clear and rational decision regarding their preferred treatment plan.

The process of securing consent in healthcare is complex, involving various stakeholders and ethical considerations. Recognizing the hierarchy of decision-makers and the ethical principles guiding consent ensures that healthcare aligns with values such as respect, beneficence, and patient-centred care. This intricate process revolves around upholding patient autonomy and well-being, which is essential in the ethical practice of medicine.

6.2 Legal Guardians and Consent

Legal guardianship, a legally defined relationship, establishes the authority of a guardian to make decisions on behalf of an incapacitated individual in healthcare matters. The legal guardian assumes the role of an advocate, prioritizing the patient's health and overall welfare. In practice, they function as surrogate decision-makers, empowered to provide consent for medical treatments, surgeries, and healthcare interventions on behalf of the incapacitated patient. This arrangement ensures that those unable to make decisions due to incapacity receive the necessary care and support while upholding ethical and legal standards.

Types of Legal Guardianship

- Parental Guardianship: Parents hold the inherent right to make healthcare decisions for their minor children, serving as their natural legal guardians unless court orders restrict or revoke these rights.

- Court-Appointed Guardians: In instances where capable parents are absent or in cases involving incapacitated adults due to mental illness, injury, or disability, the court may appoint a legal guardian. This individual could be a family member, a trusted friend, or a professional guardian.

The Consent Process with Legal Guardians

To initiate consent from legal guardians, a structured approach is followed:

- Identification and Verification of Legal Guardians: Healthcare professionals begin by confirming who holds legal guardianship over the patient. Usually, it's the parents of minors unless specified by a court order. If court-appointed, legal documents or statements are reviewed for verification.

- Communication and Information Sharing: Once identified, healthcare providers share comprehensive details about the proposed treatment. They outline risks, benefits, and alternatives, empowering informed decision-making by the guardian.

- Consent Process: Legal guardians then provide consent for the proposed medical procedure. This involves signing formal consent forms provided by the healthcare facility, affirming their understanding and agreement on behalf of the patient.

- Documentation and Records: After obtaining consent, healthcare providers meticulously document the process in the patient's medical records. This includes the guardian's identity, treatment specifics, and the consent date.

Navigating the Intersection of Legal Guardianship and Patient's Best Interests

Legal guardianship, although conferring decision-making authority, must be exercised with a paramount focus on the patient's welfare and devoid of conflicts of interest. Instances of familial disagreement or doubts regarding the guardian's choices introduce legal and ethical complexities.

Intricate legal and emotional challenges often ensue in scenarios involving disputes over guardianship or concerns about the guardian's decisions. These legal battles, particularly prevalent in complex familial situations with elderly individuals, can be emotionally draining and legally complicated.

Addressing these concerns typically involves mediation, court intervention, and the possibility of reassigning guardianship in cases of neglect or abuse, thus reinforcing the importance of upholding both legal mandates and ethical principles.

The landscape of legal guardianship in healthcare is undergoing significant changes, propelled by technological advancements and an ageing demographic. This shift is accompanied by evolving conversations about the autonomy of individuals with disabilities, pushing for a reexamination of guardianship frameworks. Legal guardians play a pivotal role in healthcare, particularly for those unable to independently make medical decisions. Recognizing the various forms of guardianship, the consent acquisition process, and the pertinent legal and ethical aspects becomes crucial for healthcare practitioners, legal experts, and society overall. These elements form the backbone of ensuring proper care and treatment for those reliant on guardianship structures in the healthcare sphere.

6.3 Healthcare Proxies and Advance Directives

Healthcare proxies and advance directives play pivotal roles in the landscape of modern healthcare, addressing critical decision-making processes when individuals are unable to advocate for themselves due to incapacity or illness. These legal documents are designed to ensure that an individual's preferences for medical treatment and care are respected and followed, even if they are unable to communicate these preferences at a later stage.

A healthcare proxy, also known as a healthcare power of attorney or a medical power of attorney, is a legal document that appoints an individual (the representative or agent) to make medical decisions on behalf of another person (the principal) in the event they are unable to make those decisions themselves. This appointed proxy has the authority to ensure that the principal's wishes regarding medical treatment and care are followed.

Imagine an elderly individual, Sarah, who faces a sudden stroke, rendering her incapable of making medical decisions. Sarah, however, had designated her daughter, Emily, as her healthcare proxy. Emily, as per the directives outlined by Sarah in advance, collaborates with healthcare professionals to make decisions aligned with Sarah's wishes. This can range from consenting to specific treatments, deciding on surgery, or choosing palliative care based on prior discussions and directives.

Advance Directives: Guiding Lights in Medical Decision-Making

Advance directives legal documents allowing individuals to outline healthcare preferences in advance serve as crucial guides in medical decision-making. These documents, encompassing living wills or medical power of attorney, offer directives on preferred medical care, particularly when the individual is incapacitated.

Consider the case of Mark, who was diagnosed with a terminal illness. Mark's living will explicitly outline his wish to forego aggressive medical interventions and opt for palliative care in case of health decline. If Mark becomes unable to articulate his preferences due to his illness, his advance directive stands as a compass for healthcare providers and his appointed proxy. This ensures that his predetermined wishes are upheld and respected.

Honouring Patient Wishes in Incapacity

In situations where a person is unable to express their medical preferences, proxies and advance directives serve to honour their choices regarding healthcare.

Healthcare providers are obligated by both legal mandates and ethical principles to uphold advance directives and decisions made by assigned proxies. However, these decisions must align with documented wishes while maintaining compliance with medical ethics and legal frameworks.

Implementing advance directives can present difficulties, particularly in intricate medical scenarios where the directives might not explicitly cover every possible situation. For instance, a directive might not encompass a novel treatment or a recently developed medical technology, leading to decision-making complexities in healthcare.

Enhancing Decision-Making Processes

1. Clear Communication Effective dialogue among patients, their proxies, families, and healthcare providers is pivotal. These discussions ensure mutual understanding of the patient's preferences, thereby averting conflicts during crucial medical decisions.

2. Maintaining Updated Directives Regular review and timely updates of advance directives are critical. Health fluctuations, novel treatments, or shifts in personal choices necessitate accurate documentation to align with the patient's current wishes.

When patients cannot communicate their preferences, having accurately documented directives becomes fundamental. These actions streamline decision-making, ensuring patients' wishes are upheld, even in their absence or incapacity.

6.4 Next of Kin and Family Consent

Navigating the complexities of healthcare decisions involves a deep understanding of the role and significance of the "next of kin." This designation carries legal, cultural, and ethical weight, particularly in pivotal medical choices and the consent process. Understanding these dimensions is crucial for ensuring the best possible outcomes in healthcare decision-making.

Legal and Cultural Contexts:

The "next of kin" concept is multifaceted, shaped by diverse legal and cultural nuances worldwide. This designation typically refers to the individual closest to the patient, legally empowered to make decisions when the patient cannot. However, the specifics of this role differ globally and within legal frameworks. Generally, it commences with a spouse, followed by adult children, parents, and extended family members in a hierarchical order. Yet, these hierarchies might vary per regional laws, occasionally prioritizing legal guardians or assigned healthcare proxies. Culturally, this role's interpretation varies too; it might align with the eldest child, a close confidant, or someone outlined in formal documentation like a living will or healthcare power of attorney, reflecting diverse cultural beliefs and legal structures.

The surrogate decision-maker, typically the next of kin, assumes a vital role in consenting to medical procedures when the patient cannot communicate preferences. Their duty involves understanding the patient's values and making healthcare decisions reflecting these principles. Picture a scenario where an individual faces a severe accident, leaving them incapacitated. Urgent medical attention is imperative, yet the patient cannot provide consent due to their condition. The next of kin takes charge, making critical decisions on treatments or surgeries. Healthcare professionals rely on their judgment to act in the patient's best interest. Nonetheless, dilemmas can surface when the surrogate's choices clash with the patient's prior directives or when family members hold differing views. For example, an ethical conflict emerges if a patient's living will oppose a specific treatment, but the next of kin insists on it. This situation highlights the complexity of decision-making when multiple opinions and patient preferences intersect.

Conflicts and Challenges:

Disagreements frequently stem from varying interpretations of what constitutes the patient's 'best interest'. Such conflicts can result from family dynamics, religious beliefs, personal values, or emotional connections. In these complex situations, healthcare providers must navigate these challenges while adhering to the principles of patient autonomy and beneficence. A common source of conflict arises when there is no clear designation of a next of kin, leading to disputes among family members. This scenario can potentially delay crucial medical decisions, affecting the patient's well-being and treatment schedule. Another challenging procedure emerges when the legally recognized next of kin doesn't align with the patient's actual preferences. For instance, a patient may have strained relationships with their closest relatives and may wish someone else to make decisions on their behalf. Balancing the patient's autonomy with adherence to legal frameworks becomes a sensitive task for healthcare professionals. Furthermore, cultural differences can significantly impact decision-making. In some cultures, decision-making may involve a more communal approach, including extended family or community elders, which may contrast with Western ideals of individual autonomy in medical decision-making.

In addressing these challenges, healthcare systems often implement specific protocols to resolve conflicts and ensure ethical decision-making. When disputes arise, mediation, ethics committees, and legal counsel may be engaged to facilitate a fair and ethical decision-making process. Open communication between family members and healthcare providers can also be instrumental in resolving conflicts and ensuring the patient's wishes are upheld. Healthcare providers must exercise great care in recognizing and respecting the patient's cultural, religious, and individual values when determining the appropriate next of kin. Understanding the intricate nuances of diverse cultural perspectives on family dynamics and decision-making is paramount for delivering patient-centred care.

Furthermore, the utilization of advance directives and legally binding documents, such as living wills or healthcare proxies, plays a crucial role in clarifying a patient's wishes and designating a decision-maker, thus minimizing ambiguity in critical situations. These legal documents provide explicit guidance on the patient's preferences regarding medical care, including who should make decisions on their behalf when they are unable to do so, reinforcing the importance of respecting patient autonomy and ensuring their well-being.

Ultimately, promoting awareness and open dialogue surrounding the complexities of next of kin and family consent in healthcare is vital for ensuring that decisions made on behalf of incapacitated patients are respectful, ethical, and in line with the patient's wishes and values.

6.5 Hierarchy of Decision-Makers

The hierarchy of decision-makers is a crucial framework for safeguarding the welfare of patients who are incapable of providing consent due to factors like unconsciousness, cognitive impairment, or conditions affecting their decision-making capacity. In situations where patients cannot express their preferences, the establishment of a structured hierarchy is paramount. This framework is rooted in the principle of prioritizing the patient's best interests while upholding ethical and legal standards. When confronted with the responsibility of making crucial healthcare decisions on behalf of such patients, this hierarchy guides the process to ensure optimal care and treatment.

Order of Decision-Making Authority

a) Patient Autonomy: The primary and most influential decision-maker is the patient themselves. In situations where patients are conscious and capable of decision-making, their wishes are the guiding principle for medical interventions. Patients can express their preferences through advance directives, which outline their choices regarding future medical treatment.

Scenario: A patient, having been diagnosed with a terminal illness, has prepared an advance directive specifying their wish to avoid aggressive life-sustaining measures. In such a case, the medical team and decision-makers must honour the patient's expressed desires.

b) Legal Guardian: When the patient lacks decision-making capacity and hasn't designated a healthcare proxy, a legal guardian, typically appointed by a court, assumes the role of decision-maker. This guardian could be a family member, a professional guardian, or someone explicitly specified to make healthcare choices for the incapacitated individual.

Scenario: A patient who has suffered a severe brain injury and is in a comatose state has no previously designated healthcare proxy. In this case, the court may appoint a family member as the legal guardian to make medical decisions on behalf of the incapacitated patient.

c) Healthcare Proxy or Medical Power of Attorney: If the patient has previously designated a healthcare proxy or granted medical power of attorney, this individual becomes the primary decision-maker. This appointed proxy is entrusted to make healthcare choices based on the patient's previously expressed wishes or in their best interest.

Scenario: An individual, aware of a forthcoming surgery, designates a close friend as their healthcare proxy. During the surgery, unforeseen complications arise, rendering the patient unable to communicate. The designated proxy is then responsible for making decisions regarding the patient's treatment based on their understanding of the patient's preferences.

d) Next of Kin: In the absence of the aforementioned designated individuals or legal documents, the next of kin assumes the role of decision-maker. The next of kin is often a family member identified as the closest relation to the patient.

Scenario: In an emergency situation where there are no legal documents or appointed proxies, a patient who has been in a severe accident is unconscious and unable to provide consent. In this scenario, the medical team might look to the patient's next of kin, usually a spouse or parent, to make immediate decisions regarding the patient's medical care.

Conflict Resolution Among Decision-Makers

Conflict resolution among decision-makers, significantly when their perspectives diverge on the patient's best interests, can dramatically impact patient care. Resolving these conflicts is paramount to ensure the patient receives optimal treatment. Healthcare facilities employ mechanisms, such as mediation and ethics committees, to address such disputes. Mediation involves critical stakeholders—the medical team, family members, and legal representatives—to facilitate consensus. Additionally, ethics committees within healthcare institutions serve as forums for discussions and conflict resolution. Central to these discussions is the best interest standard, ensuring medical decisions prioritize the patient's health and well-being. Evaluating treatment options involves thoroughly assessing risks and benefits while considering the patient's values and any previously expressed wishes, if available.

Legal and Ethical Decision-Making Framework

- Legal Documents: Advance directives and living will serve as crucial legal tools, enabling individuals to outline their healthcare preferences in advance. These directives become pivotal guides when patients are unable to communicate their desires.

- Policy and Legal Influence: Laws and healthcare regulations, such as the Patient Self-Determination Act, establish the legal underpinning for decision-makers in medical contexts. They set the stage for responsibilities and the scope of decision-making.

- Ethical Guidelines: Guiding the actions of decision-makers are fundamental ethical principles. Beneficence, prioritizing the patient's best interest; autonomy, honouring the patient's choices; non-maleficence, ensuring no harm; and justice, advocating fair and equitable treatment, all play vital roles in decision-making processes within healthcare settings. These principles shape the ethical compass by which decisions are made in patient care and treatment.

While structured, the hierarchy of decision-making in healthcare encounters challenges stemming from intricate family dynamics, diverse cultures, and the evolution of medical technologies. With the advent of AI in healthcare, this landscape has become even more complex. This amalgamates legal, ethical, and medical facets to ascertain decisions that align with the patient's best interest. Understanding and honouring this hierarchical structure requires a collaborative effort among healthcare providers, legal entities, and families. This collaborative approach aims to guarantee the delivery of the most suitable care, even in the face of challenging and uncertain situations. This interplay of factors ensures that the patient's well-being remains the central focus of decision-making processes.

CHAPTER 7: VALIDITY OF CONSENTS

When discussing the term 'valid' in medical treatment consent, it's essential to differentiate between its foundational and legal aspects. This distinction, often blurred, can lead to overlooking either the foundational basis or the legal requisites. In common law, consent to treatment varies concerning 'valid consent' (or 'real consent') and 'informed consent.' The absence of valid consent might result in criminal charges like assault or civil trespass claims, while a lack of informed consent can constitute negligence. Courts gradually acknowledged the latter, considering it a well-grounded concept. A mentally sound adult holds the right to choose among available treatments, and their consent must precede any invasive procedure.

A sound basis for consent aligns with ethical principles and legal standards. It necessitates voluntariness, capacity, and adequate information. Since the Montgomery case of 2015, informed consent has been a firm element of English law, mandating that patients receive comprehensive information to make informed decisions. Neglecting this obligation could lead to negligence claims. The General Medical Council emphasizes patient education and adopts a partnership model for consent, and failure to adhere to GMC guidelines may result in charges of professional misconduct affecting a doctor's registration.

The legal concept of consent bears varying meanings, sometimes indicating a sound basis and other times referring to its legality. This duality may lead to overlooking aspects crucial to either a solid foundation or the necessary legal prerequisites. In the context of medical treatment, consent encompasses dimensions of 'valid consent' (or 'real consent') and 'informed consent' under common law. Failure to secure valid consent can result in criminal assault or a civil claim of trespass to the person, while neglecting informed consent can constitute negligence. Notably, an adult of sound mind holds the entitlement to decide on treatment options and must grant consent before any invasive procedure.

Valid consent is rooted in ethical principles and legal compliance, necessitating voluntariness, capacity, and adequate information. Following the landmark case of Montgomery in 2015, informed consent became an integral part of English law. Patients must receive the necessary information to make informed decisions, failure of which could prompt negligence claims. The General Medical Council (GMC) emphasizes informed consent, promoting a partnership model between patients and practitioners. However, legislative measures can adjust these requirements, exemplified by regulations like the EU Clinical Trials Regulation 536/2014, which explicitly mandates informed consent for clinical trials, albeit not yet in effect. The complexities of consent, both legally and ethically, navigate a delicate balance between autonomy and legal compliance, shaping the landscape of medical practices and patient rights.

Validity of Consent for Minors

- **Emancipated Minor's Rights:** This section doesn't restrict an emancipated minor's rights to consent to health services or control access to protected health care information according to applicable law.

- **Criteria for Minor Consent:** Minors can provide consent for health services or control access to health care information under specific conditions:

- **Marital, Parental, or Educational Status:** Minors claiming marriage, parenthood, or high school graduation.

- **Independent Living:** Minors separated from parents/legal guardians and self-supporting.

- **Health Conditions:** Minors pregnant, with reportable communicable diseases, including STDs, or facing drug/substance abuse issues.

- **Scope of Self-Consent:** Self-consent is applicable only for preventing, diagnosing, and treating these conditions.

- **Responsibilities of Health Professionals:** Professionals accepting responsibility for treatment must counsel or refer the minor for counselling regarding pregnancy, STDs, or substance abuse.

- **Emergency Care:** Minors needing emergency care that is crucial for their health can consent. Parents/guardians should be informed unless exceptional circumstances exist.

- **Consent for Child's Health Services:** A minor who has a child can consent to health services for the child.

- **Consent for Spouse's Health Services:** A minor can consent to their spouse's health services if the spouse can't consent due to physical or mental incapacity.

Validity of Consent for Married Couples:

- **Parties Eligible to Provide Consent:** Married couples, both Emirati and international, are eligible to provide consent for healthcare decisions.

- **Treatment Authorization:** Consent for some selected medical procedures requires joint agreement from both spouses, ensuring mutual authorization for healthcare actions.

- **Specific Conditions for Consent:** Both partners should meet certain conditions, such as being officially married with documented proof or having undergone a minimum period of attempting pregnancy.

- **Medical Criteria for Consent for infertility treatments:** The couples must satisfy medical criteria indicating infertility or the necessity for assisted reproductive techniques.

- **Permissible Treatments:** The authorized consent allows access to a range of treatments such as In Vitro Fertilization (IVF), Gamete Intrafallopian Transfer (GIFT), and other established fertilization techniques outlined by the Oversight and Control Committee.

- **Prohibited Actions:** Certain medical procedures like Gestational Surrogacy or Embryo Donation remain prohibited by law and are not encompassed under the consent of married couples for healthcare treatments in certain jurisdictions.

Validity of Consent for Elders:

- **Competency of Consent:** Elderly individuals must exhibit mental capacity to comprehend and make decisions about their healthcare.

- **Information and Understanding:** They should receive comprehensive details regarding proposed treatments, potential risks, success rates, and alternative options in a manner that they can understand.

- **Freedom of Choice:** Elders must be able to make decisions without coercion or pressure, ensuring their consent is voluntary.

- **Proxy Consent:** If an elder lacks capacity, a legally authorized representative, often a family member or legal guardian, can provide consent on their behalf.

- **Healthcare Directives:** Advance directives or living wills legally document an elder's preferences for healthcare decisions if they become incapacitated.

- **Medical Power of Attorney:** Designating a healthcare proxy empowers someone to make healthcare choices when the elder cannot.

- **Legal Framework:** Laws regarding consent for elders vary by region, ensuring compliance with legal requirements while respecting an elder's autonomy and dignity in healthcare decisions.

7.1 Guidance Distinguishing Between Valid And Informed Consent

Numerous guidelines outline consent requirements at common law, varying in their approach. Some delineate the legal distinction as stated earlier, while others encompass pertinent legal and ethical principles. Specific guidelines emphasize the necessity for patients to be thoroughly informed about risks and alternatives to obtain valid consent. For instance, the Department of Health's 2009 guidance acknowledges that any touch without valid consent could amount to the civil or criminal offence of battery. This guidance highlights the crucial aspect of receiving adequate information, encompassing both the validity and sufficiency of the details provided for making an informed decision (Department of Health, 2009, p. 5). Exploring these different approaches offers insights into the complexities surrounding the criteria for obtaining valid consent.

To grant valid consent, a clear comprehension of the procedure's nature and objectives is crucial. Any distortion of these aspects can nullify the consent. While detailing the procedure's nature and aims ensures valid consent in terms of potential claims of battery, meeting the legal duty of care requires more. Negligence claims might arise if essential information beyond the procedure's basics isn't provided, leading to harm resulting from the treatment received. Thus, simply outlining the nature and purpose of a procedure isn't exhaustive in meeting the practitioner's duty of care under the law.

The Care Quality Commission, guided by Regulation 11 of the Health and Social Care Act 2008 (Regulated Activities) Regulations 2014, insists on consent as a prerequisite for providing care under its brief guidance. This consent hinges on adequate information, necessitating a comprehensive understanding of risks and alternatives. Meanwhile, the GMC offers extensive guidance on consent, covering capacity, voluntariness, and sufficient information, without delineating between battery and negligence laws. However, while acknowledging the potential invalidity of involuntary consent or refusal of essential information, the GMC's brief mention of validity lacks clarification on what truly constitutes valid consent, raising questions about its practical utility.

The National Health Service (NHS) guidelines assert that valid consent necessitates voluntariness, informed decision-making, and capacity to decide. Legally, this holds true, emphasizing that informed consent entails comprehensive information on the treatment, including risks, benefits, alternatives, and potential outcomes of non-treatment. However, as previously discussed, while informed consent demands extensive details, validity necessitates only fundamental information, not a comprehensive understanding of risks, benefits, and alternatives. Consequently, when examined in isolation, these statements are legally accurate, but when considered together as components of valid consent, the NHS definition of 'informed' for the purpose of validating consent falls short.

In essence, for consent to hold validity:

- Firstly, the patient needs to be competent, possessing the mental capacity to comprehend the given information. Without adequate information, patients cannot make informed decisions about their treatment. This information should encompass a comprehensive explanation of the investigation, diagnosis, or treatment, as well as the associated probabilities of success, risks of failure, or harm linked with various treatment options.

- Secondly, the patient must be capable of freely giving their consent without any external coercion or undue influence. These criteria establish the foundation for ensuring that consent is well-informed and provided voluntarily, maintaining the patient's autonomy in decision-making.

The core elements of competency, adequate information, and voluntary consent are crucial aspects defining valid consent. However, the delineation of sufficient information varies across guidelines, making it an imprecise marker for validating consent. Institutions like the General Dental Council distinguish between valid and informed consent, acknowledging that the latter might not encapsulate all components of valid consent—namely, voluntariness and capacity—yet they incorporate the essence of informed consent within the broader concept of valid consent. Similarly, the Royal College of Obstetricians and Gynaecologists outlines legal prerequisites for informed consent within their 2015 guidelines on 'Obtaining valid consent.' Meanwhile, the General Optical Council's guidance on 'Obtaining valid consent' acknowledges the multifaceted nature of consent, suggesting a necessity beyond basic information to avert any potential battery claims. These distinctions underscore the nuanced interpretations and applications of valid consent within professional regulations.

7.2 Legal Distinction - Does the label matter?

Professional guidance rightly demands both valid and informed consent, aligning with legal requirements. While some argue that using "valid consent" lacks legal precision, legality doesn't exclusively define the term 'valid.' Yet, treatment should be withheld if consent lacks ethical validity despite meeting legal standards. Thus, clarifying that uninformed consent lacks validity ethically holds merit. However, these guidelines often lack clarity on the ethical, not just the legal stance, potentially causing confusion, compounded by discrepancies among guidelines. This distinction holds practical significance beyond theory, warranting precise delineation within professional directives. Consequently, bridging this gap is imperative to ensure a unified, comprehensive understanding of consent's ethical and legal dimensions.

Lords Kerr and Reed's perspective in Montgomery delineates patients' entitlement to opt out of information concerning risks, benefits, and alternatives, emphasizing the crucial role of patient consent. Conversely, in the context of medical procedures, the absence of fundamental information renders the consent invalid, such as a patient undergoing a proposed operation on their left leg without being informed and agreeing to it. A misunderstanding by healthcare professionals (HCPs) regarding this stance may lead to two distinct issues.

One scenario involves HCPs insisting on disclosing material risks despite the patient's explicit refusal to receive such information out of concern for consent validity. This approach disregards patient autonomy and potentially exposes them to harm. Conversely, another situation arises when a patient declines unnecessary details, leading HCPs to withhold even basic information about the proposed procedure, thereby compromising the validity of consent and denying patient autonomy. Negligence may occur if disclosed information causes harm, while a lack of disclosure may constitute battery. The guidance provided, including that from the General Medical Council (GMC), lacks clarity in avoiding these pitfalls. Medical Protection advises disclosure of risks even against a patient's wishes to align with perceived consent requirements. While the GMC acknowledges that refusal of basic information may invalidate consent, it falls short in elucidating valid consent requirements and their consequences.

The concept of the 'therapeutic exception' in negligence is crucial, allowing for the withholding of material risks disclosure if it poses serious harm to the patient. However, its application to the tort of battery remains uncertain. This ambiguity may result in healthcare professionals (HCPs) refraining from sharing fundamental information with patients, fearing potential harm. Such confusion could lead to unintended consequences, impacting patient-provider trust and comprehensive medical understanding. Clarifying the boundaries of this exception is imperative to ensure transparent communication between HCPs and patients.

The Mental Capacity Act 2005 (British Legislation) introduction prompts inquiry into the expanded scope of informational requirements beyond mere 'basic information.' Section 2 outlines that individuals with a mind or brain impairment may lack capacity under section 3 if they cannot comprehend, retain, use, weigh information, or communicate decisions despite reasonable facilitation attempts (section 1 (3)). Clarity emerges on the necessary comprehension level—where an inability to grasp material risks impedes decision-making, indicating a capacity deficit. However, capacity doesn't mandate a comprehensive understanding of such risks (section 1 (2)). Negligence might govern legal actions if someone consents without grasping material risks; lacking capacity could lead to a battery lawsuit due to invalid consent. Understanding the 'salient details' suffices for decision-making, permitting capacity even if peripheral information eludes comprehension. Overemphasizing the need for total risk comprehension could unjustly heighten capacity standards for those meeting incapacity criteria.

The essence of informed consent hinges on its voluntary and capacitous nature. However, mere validity does not guarantee adequate information exchange. The variance in informational thresholds between battery and negligence delineates this distinction. Regrettably, this nuance often remains obscured in the abundance of consent-related directives. Not every guideline necessitates an exhaustive delineation of the legal disparity between battery and negligence. Frequently, fundamental guidance serves as a touchstone for patients' expectations and healthcare practitioners' obligations when obtaining consent. This rudimentary framework sidesteps delving into the validity concept. Nonetheless, comprehensive directives, such as those from the GMC, warrant a deeper exploration of the dichotomy between valid and informed consent. The absence of this exploration risks generating conflicting or ambiguous directives. Moreover, it might spur misinterpretations that elevate capacity thresholds, mandate unwanted information provision to patients, or withhold even essential details from capable patients who opt not to delve deeper, potentially causing serious harm based on healthcare professionals' assumptions.

7.3 Navigating Consent in Healthcare: Understanding AND and AMA

In healthcare, consent is critical in decision-making, notably in delicate areas such as Allowing Natural Death (AND) and Against Medical Advice (AMA). These terms encapsulate intricate ethical, legal, and medical considerations, delineating the boundaries between patient autonomy and healthcare provider responsibilities. AND signifies a patient's choice to forgo or withdraw medical interventions when further treatment may only prolong the dying process without offering realistic chances of recovery. Rooted in the principle of honouring a patient's wishes and dignity, AND aligns with their values and preferences regarding end-of-life care, especially in terminal or vegetative states where interventions might amplify suffering without enhancing life quality. The process involves comprehensive discussions among the healthcare team, the patient, and their family, ensuring clear comprehension and respect for the patient's desires. It necessitates obtaining informed consent, elucidating the prognosis, treatment options, and associated risks, and enabling informed decision-making. At its core, AND rests on patient autonomy, recognizing their right to decide, even if it implies refusing treatment while necessitating appropriate palliative care to ensure comfort.

Conversely, Against Medical Advice (AMA) denotes situations where a patient rejects recommended treatment or leaves a healthcare facility against professional advice. This decision could stem from personal beliefs, distrust, or alternative treatment preferences. Legally and ethically, the AMA raises concerns, obliging healthcare providers to ensure patients fully grasp the ramifications of their choice, including worsening conditions or potential complications. Rigorous documentation becomes pivotal to mitigating legal liabilities, emphasizing the significance of patient comprehension and decision-making. Efforts encourage patients to reconsider by addressing concerns, educating them, and exploring alternative options in line with their preferences. The fundamental disparity between AND and AMA lies in the decision-making process: while AND involves collaborative decisions honouring a patient's end-of-life care wishes, AMA represents a unilateral choice against medical advice, potentially conflicting with healthcare providers' recommendations.

Both scenarios highlight the vital role of informed consent, empowering patients with comprehensive understanding of their condition, treatment options, and potential outcomes. It fosters patient participation in decision-making, advocating autonomy and patient-centred care. Healthcare professionals navigating these scenarios must do so with empathy, recognizing the legal and ethical intricacies. Respecting patient autonomy while prioritizing their well-being remains paramount, whether honouring a patient's choice in end-of-life care or addressing concerns when they go against medical advice. In summary, AND and AMA underscore the nuances of consent in healthcare, emphasizing the essence of informed consent, patient autonomy, and balancing patient preferences with ethical considerations. Healthcare providers must approach these scenarios sensitively, emphasizing communication and adherence to ethical principles while honouring patient choices.

Legal and Ethical Aspects of Consent in the UAE

- Article (3) of the UAE Medical Liability Law mandates that all professional practitioners uphold their work responsibilities with precision and integrity, adhering to established scientific and technical norms and ensuring patient care. Exploiting patients' needs for personal gain or any form of discrimination among patients is strictly prohibited, and practitioners are obligated to comply with the state's relevant laws.

- Article (4), in addition to the overarching legal requirements, specifies the obligations incumbent upon physicians. These include adherence to professional rules pertinent to their degree and specialization; thorough documentation of a patient's health status and medical history; utilization of appropriate diagnostic and treatment tools; diligent use of medical equipment in line with established scientific principles; informing patients about available medication options; precise prescription details; disclosure of the nature and severity of an illness unless it contradicts the patient's interest or emotional readiness; notification of next of kin or relatives under specific circumstances; informing patients or their families about potential complications arising from treatment and offering necessary care; collaboration with other physicians and healthcare professionals involved in a patient's care; and reporting suspected cases of communicable diseases according to legislative protocols. These stringent guidelines emphasize transparency, patient involvement, and interdisciplinary cooperation for effective and ethical medical practice.

- Article (5) delineates the obligations of a physician, outlining a set of actions that are strictly prohibited. Firstly, the administration of treatment without the explicit consent of the patient is forbidden, except under emergency circumstances where obtaining consent is unfeasible or when dealing with a contagious disease that poses a threat to public health. However, concerning examinations, diagnosis, and the initial administration of medication, consent from an incapacitated patient is permissible, with a condition to inform the patient's relatives or associates about the treatment plan. Furthermore, it is mandatory for a physician to offer treatment or initial aid to an injured individual within their expertise. If the case exceeds their specialization, the physician should provide preliminary assistance and subsequently refer the patient to a specialist or the nearest medical facility, as per the patient's preference. Additionally, employing unauthorized or illegal methods in treating a patient is strictly prohibited. Lastly, prescribing any treatment without conducting a clinical examination of the patient is deemed inappropriate. Notably, Health Authorities are empowered to establish a telehealth system adhering to the specified regulations within this Decree-Law.

- Article (6) defines a medical error as any mistake made by a Professional Practitioner for various reasons: lack of technical knowledge common to professionals of the same degree and specialization, failure to adhere to established professional and medical principles, lack of due diligence, and negligence. The criteria for categorizing a severe medical error will be outlined in the executive regulations of this Decree-Law.

- Article (7) outlines the parameters for Sex Reassignment Surgeries (Sex correction) governed by specific controls: Firstly, when an individual's gender identity is ambiguous and warrants clarification regarding their male or female identity. Secondly, when an individual possesses sexual and physical attributes inconsistent with their physiological, biological, and genetic characteristics. Verification of these conditions outlined in Paragraphs (1 and 2) necessitates substantiation through medical reports and approval by a specialized medical committee, formed by the Health Authority. This committee's role involves defining the patient's gender identity and authorizing the reassignment surgery, with an additional step of referring the case to a psychologist for necessary psychological preparation.

- Article (8) outlines strict conditions for surgical interventions, with exceptions for immediate life-saving or complication-averting emergencies. For surgeries to proceed: a) The performing physician must hold suitable qualifications, including academic expertise and precise surgical skills. b) Comprehensive tests must confirm the necessity and suitability of the surgery based on the patient's health condition. c) Written consent from legally competent patients or from relatives up to the fourth degree for partially or wholly incompetent patients is required, with informative disclosure of potential complications. d) In cases where consent is unattainable, a detailed report endorsed by the attending physician, another facility physician, and the facility manager may suffice, except for legally competent patients without possible consent sources. e) Surgeries must be conducted in well-equipped healthcare centers. The Decree-Law's executive regulations cover additional specifications for specialized treatment cases.

- Article (9) stipulates conditions for discharging patients from health facilities. Firstly, discharge hinges upon the patient's health status, aligning with recognized medical standards. Additionally, discharge to another facility for continued treatment requires ensuring the patient's safety during transfer and compliance with medical protocols. Should a competent patient request discharge against medical advice, they must be fully informed of potential consequences and sign a written acknowledgment. For partially or thoroughly incompetent patients, transfer necessitates written approval from a facility physician endorsed by their guardian. Lastly, individuals staying in the facility without medical reasons should leave upon request.

- Article (10) strictly prohibits terminating a patient's life under any circumstance, even at the explicit request of the patient, guardian, or custodian. Furthermore, removal of Cardiopulmonary Resuscitation (CPR) equipment is prohibited except in cases of cardiopulmonary arrest or when all brain functions cease entirely, based on precise medical criteria stipulated by a decision from the Minister. This decision must align with the determination made by physicians that the arrest is irreversible.

- Article (11) outlines the circumstances allowing for natural death through the non-application of CPR when a patient is in a terminal state, based on several criteria. These include cases where the patient suffers from an incurable illness and has exhausted all available treatment options and when medical evidence shows the futility of further interventions. Additionally, the attending physician's recommendation against CPR and a consensus among a minimum of three consultant physicians supporting the cessation of CPR constitute further grounds. In these situations, consent from the patient, guardian, or custodian is not mandatory. However, it's crucial to note that withholding it is not permissible if the patient explicitly requests CPR, even if considered futile.

- Article (12) prohibits the creation of human cloning and any associated research or experiments aimed at its development. It mandates that medical research or experiments involving individuals can only proceed with their explicit consent and written permission from the designated authority as outlined in the executive regulations. This ensures ethical considerations and proper oversight for medical studies involving human subjects, safeguarding their rights and well-being.

- Article (13) stipulates that the implantation of artificial organs within the body must only occur after verifying their suitability and safety for the patient and preparing the body to accept these artificial implants. This crucial directive underscores the necessity for ensuring the compatibility and innocuousness of these artificial organs with the recipient's body before any such procedure takes place.

- Article (14) stipulates that employing assisted reproductive technology or implanting an embryo within a woman's uterus is permissible exclusively for legally married couples and upon their explicit written consent. This practice is strictly limited to the context of their lawful marital union.

- Article (15) strictly prohibits any reproductive regulation action or intervention without both spouses' explicit request or consent. Additionally, sterilizing a woman is only permissible when a medical specialized committee, consisting of at least three physicians, unanimously determines that pregnancy or delivery will undoubtedly endanger the mother's life. In such cases, the procedure can proceed solely with the wife's written consent after informing the husband about the decision and gaining his awareness of the situation.

Medical Consents in the UAE and globally have evolved significantly over the years, reflecting changes in medical ethics, legal frameworks, and societal norms. In the United Arab Emirates (UAE), medical consent is governed by federal laws that emphasize patient autonomy and the right to make informed decisions about their healthcare. The UAE has made strides in aligning its regulations with international standards, ensuring that patients are adequately informed about their treatment options and potential risks. Globally, medical consent practices vary widely, influenced by cultural, religious, and legal factors. In some countries, such as the United States and European nations, informed consent is a cornerstone of medical practice, requiring healthcare providers to communicate effectively with patients and obtain their explicit permission before proceeding with treatment. However, challenges persist in ensuring universal access to comprehensive information and fostering true patient empowerment in the decision-making process. As a rule, the author recommends obtaining a written consent, whenever permissible to safeguard yourself against future medicolegal claims.

Remember, there is no specific time limit for obtaining consent in advance. Some regulatory recommend thirty days as the time limit for procedure consents, however, Patients may have additional questions or develop doubts about their decision during the waiting period. It's important to reconfirm consent before the procedure, providing an opportunity to address any further queries from the patient. Documentation of the confirmed consent should be included in the patient's medical record or as a supplementary note on the original consent form, signed and dated.

As technology advances and healthcare becomes increasingly complex, the issue of medical consents will continue to be a critical aspect of healthcare delivery worldwide. It is imperative for healthcare systems to prioritize transparency, communication, and respect for patient autonomy to uphold ethical standards and promote trust between patients and providers on a global scale.

In conclusion, the landscape of medical consents underscores the importance of respecting patient autonomy and promoting informed decision-making in healthcare settings. While progress has been made in enhancing legal frameworks and ethical practices surrounding medical consents, there remain challenges in ensuring universal adherence to these principles across different cultural contexts. Moving forward, it is essential for healthcare systems to prioritize patient education, communication, and empowerment to foster a culture of trust and collaboration between patients and providers.

References

(2024). Google.com. https://www.ehs.gov.ae/app_content/legislations/php-law-en-30/mobile/index.html#p=1

Ali, F., Gopi Gajera, Gowda, G. S., Preeti Srinivasa, & Mahesh Gowda. (2019a). Consent in current psychiatric practice and research: An Indian perspective. *Indian Journal of Psychiatry*, *61*(10), 667. https://doi.org/10.4103/psychiatry.IndianJPsychiatry_163_19

American Medical Association. (n.d.-a). *Consent, Communication & Decision Making | ama-coe*. Code-Medical-Ethics.ama-Assn.org. https://code-medical-ethics.ama-assn.org/chapters/consent-communication-decision-making

American Medical Association. (n.d.-c). *Informed Consent | ama-coe*. Code-Medical-Ethics.ama-Assn.org. https://code-medical-ethics.ama-assn.org/ethics-opinions/informed-consent

Bazzano, L. A., Durant, J., & Brantley, P. R. (2021f). A Modern History of Informed Consent and the Role of Key Information. *The Ochsner Journal*, *21*(1), 81–85. https://doi.org/10.31486/toj.19.0105

Bramstedt, K. A. (2003a). Questioning the decision-making capacity of surrogates. *Internal Medicine Journal*, *33*(5-6), 257–259. https://doi.org/10.1046/j.1445-5994.2003.00386.x

Commissioner, O. of the. (2019b, February 8). *Informed Consent for Clinical Trials*. FDA. https://www.fda.gov/patients/clinical-trials-what-patients-need-know/informed-consent-clinical-

trials#:~:text=This%20information%20is%20provided%
20to

Competence and Informed Consent | Saint Joseph's University.
(n.d.-a). Www.sju.edu.
https://www.sju.edu/centers/icb/blog/competence-and-
informed-consent#:~:text=An%20adult%20patient

Consent Forms. (n.d.-b). Fertility and Reproductive Medicine.
Retrieved May 31, 2024, from
https://fertility.nm.org/consent-forms.html

Gambhir, R. S., Singh, S., Kaur, A., Nanda, T., & Kakar, H.
(2014a). Informed consent: Corner stone in ethical
medical and dental practice. *Journal of Family Medicine
and Primary Care, 3*(1), 68.
https://doi.org/10.4103/2249-4863.130284

Ghooi, R. B. (2011a). The Nuremberg Code - A Critique.
Perspectives in Clinical Research, 2(2), 72.
https://doi.org/10.4103/2229-3485.80371

Ghooi, R. B. (2011b). The Nuremberg Code - A Critique.
Perspectives in Clinical Research, 2(2), 72.
https://doi.org/10.4103/2229-3485.80371

*Guardianship : Ministry of Social Justice and Empowerment
(MSJE).* (n.d.-a). Thenationaltrust.gov.in. Retrieved May
31, 2024, from
https://thenationaltrust.gov.in/content/innerpage/guardia
nship.php#:~:text=In%20the%20case%20of%20a

*GUIDELINES FOR PATIENT CONSENT Guidelines for
Patient Consent.* (n.d.-b).
https://www.dha.gov.ae/uploads/112021/51f61916-
2c36-435a-9ed1-a406b9739cec.pdf

Gupta, U. C. (2013a). Informed Consent in Clinical research:
Revisiting Few Concepts and Areas. *Perspectives in*

Clinical Research, 4(1), 26–32.
https://doi.org/10.4103/2229-3485.106373

Hall, D. E., Prochazka, A. V., & Fink, A. S. (2012b). Informed consent for clinical treatment. *Canadian Medical Association Journal*, 184(5), 533–540. https://doi.org/10.1503/cmaj.112120

Informed Consent in Pediatric Patients | OncoLink. (n.d.-a). Www.oncolink.org. Retrieved May 31, 2024, from https://www.oncolink.org/cancers/pediatric/resources/inf ormed-consent-in-pediatric-patients#:~:text=Who%20makes%20decisions%20for%20children

Informed Consent: I. History of Informed Consent | Encyclopedia.com. (2019b). Encyclopedia.com. https://www.encyclopedia.com/science/encyclopedias-almanacs-transcripts-and-maps/informed-consent-i-history-informed-consent

Jackson, E. (2021a). Challenging the comparison in montgomery between patients and "consumers exercising choices." *Medical Law Review*, 29(4). https://doi.org/10.1093/medlaw/fwab031

Kumar, N. (2013b). Informed consent: Past and present. *Perspectives in Clinical Research*, 4(1), 21. https://doi.org/10.4103/2229-3485.106372

Nandimath, O. (2009a). Consent and medical treatment: The legal paradigm in India. *Indian Journal of Urology*, 25(3), 343. https://doi.org/10.4103/0970-1591.56202

National Institute on Aging. (2022b). *Advance care planning: Advance directives for health care.* https://www.nia.nih.gov/health/advance-care-planning/advance-care-planning-advance-directives-health-care

O'shea, T. (n.d.-a). *The Essex Autonomy Project CONSENT IN HISTORY, THEORY AND PRACTICE.* https://autonomy.essex.ac.uk/wp-content/uploads/2016/11/Consent-GPR-June-2012.pdf

Shah, P., Thornton, I., Turrin, D., & Hipskind, J. E. (2023d). *Informed consent.* National Library of Medicine; StatPearls Publishing. https://www.ncbi.nlm.nih.gov/books/NBK430827/

The History of the Informed Consent Requirement in United States Federal Policy. (n.d.-a). https://dash.harvard.edu/bitstream/handle/1/8852197/Wandler.pdf?sequence=1

What (and Who) Is Next of Kin, and Why Does It Matter? (n.d.-a). Investopedia. Retrieved May 31, 2024, from https://www.investopedia.com/terms/n/next-of-kin.asp#:~:text=Take%20a%20situation%20where%20someone

Wikipedia Contributors. (2018b, December 9). *Doctors' trial.* Wikipedia; Wikimedia Foundation. https://en.wikipedia.org/wiki/Doctors%27_trial

Wikipedia Contributors. (2019a, January 24). *Implied consent.* Wikipedia; Wikimedia Foundation. https://en.wikipedia.org/wiki/Implied_consent

Zohny, H. (2020a, November 27). *Why do we need to distinguish "valid" and "informed" consent to medical treatment?* Journal of Medical Ethics Blog. https://blogs.bmj.com/medical-ethics/2020/11/27/why-do-we-need-to-distinguish-valid-and-informed-consent-to-medical-

treatment/#:~:text=So%20if%20the%20consenting%20p
atient

MOHAP; 2016,
https://mohap.gov.ae/assets/6df06005/Ministerial%20Re
solution%20No.%201448%20of%202017%20On%20A
doption%20of%20Code%20of%20Ethics%20and%20Pr
ofessional%20Conduct%20for%20Health%20Profession
als_637910546760048033_638187983294940621.pdf.as
px

Verses Kindler Publication

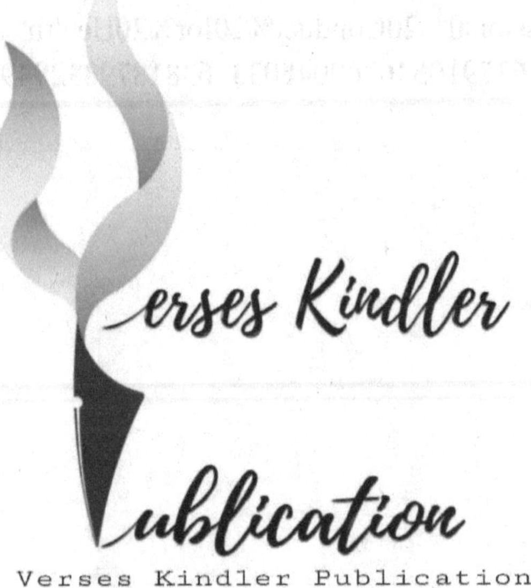

Reach us through our website -

https://www.verseskindlerpublication.com/

For more information visit our Instagram or Facebook page.